SELF-ASSESSMENT OF

CURRENT KNOWLEDGE

IN

INFECTIOUS DISEASES

By

RICHARD V. McCLOSKEY, M.D.

Head, Section of Infectious Diseases
Department of Medicine
Albert Einstein Medical Center
Daroff Division
Philadelphia, Pennsylvania

Formerly

Professor of Medicine
Head, Section of Infectious Diseases
University of Texas Medical School
at San Antonio
San Antonio, Texas

RC 111
M23
1972

1241 Multiple Choice Questions
and Referenced Answers

MEDICAL EXAMINATION PUBLISHING COMPANY, INC.

65-36 Fresh Meadow Lane

Flushing, N.Y. 11365

1972

285668

Library of Congress
Catalog Card Number

78-160718

ISBN   0-87488-263-X

November 1972

INTRODUCTION

A variety of question formats have been used to aid the reader in reviewing currently published information relating to bacteriology, virology, tuberculosis, mycology, parasitology, diagnostic microbiology and antimicrobial therapy. The data reviewed apply to both adult and pediatric infectious diseases, as well as the basic sciences applicable to these clinical specialties. Case histories are used to illustrate epidemiology, clinical presentations, and therapy. Almost all of the articles reviewed have been published between 1969 and 1972, in an effort to emphasize the *current* knowledge applicable to infectious diseases. The author wishes to express his gratitude to William Jackson and Joyce Taylor for their support.

What one fool can do, another can.
(Ancient Simian proverb)

Richard McCloskey, M.D.

SELF-ASSESSMENT OF CURRENT KNOWLEDGE IN INFECTIOUS DISEASES

TABLE OF CONTENTS

SECTION

I   BACTERIOLOGY
Questions 1-322   7

II   VIROLOGY
Questions 323-498   40

III   MYCOLÓGY - TUBERCULOSIS
Questions 499-623   56

IV   ANTIMICROBIAL AGENTS AND THERAPY
Questions 624-908   72

V   PARASITIC DISEASES
Questions 909-966   104

VI   IMMUNOLOGY AND PHYSIOLOGY
Questions 967-1069   110

VII   CASE HISTORIES
Questions 1070-1203   124

VIII   DIFFERENTIAL DIAGNOSIS
Questions 1204-1241   155

ANSWER KEY   160

FOR EACH OF THE FOLLOWING MULTIPLE CHOICE QUESTIONS,
SELECT THE ONE MOST APPROPRIATE ANSWER:

1. THE MOST COMMON SITE OF INFECTION IN PATIENTS WITH
MULTIPLE MYELOMA ADMITTED TO THE HOSPITAL BECAUSE OF
INFECTION IS:
A. Skin
B. Urinary tract
C. Lung
D. Sepsis
E. Peritonitis

Ref. Meyers, B. R., Hirshman, S. Z., Axelrod, J.: Current Patterns of
Infection in Multiple Myeloma. Amer J Med, 52:87, 1972.

2. WHICH OF THE FOLLOWING HAS BEEN DEMONSTRATED TO
SIGNIFICANTLY REDUCE MORTALITY IN ALL CASES IN THE TREAT-
MENT OF CLOSTRIDIUM PERFRINGENS ABORTION WITH INTRA-
VASCULAR HEMOLYSIS?:
A. Heparinization
B. Uterine curettage
C. Hysterectomy
D. Hyperbaric therapy
E. None of the above

Ref. Pritchard, J. A., Whalley, P. J.: Abortion Complicated by
Clostridium Perfringens Infection. Am J Obst Gynec, 111:484, 1971.

3. THE PERCENTAGE OF NEONATES WITH SEPTICEMIA IN WHOM
A SINGLE BLOOD CULTURE CAN BE EXPECTED TO BE POSITIVE IS:
A. Less than 1%
B. 20%
C. 5%
D. Nearly 100%
E. 50%

Ref. Granciosi, R. A., Favara, B. E.: Single Blood Culture for Con-
firmation of Diagnosis of Neonatal Septicemia. Am J Clin Pathol,
57:215, 1972.

4. THE ORGANISM MOST COMMONLY ISOLATED BY TYMPANOPARA-
CENTESIS FROM OTITIS MEDIA, OCCURRING DURING THE FIRST 6
WEEKS OF LIFE, IS:
A. H. influenzae
B. Proteus species
C. D. pneumoniae
D. S. viridans
E. E. coli

Ref. Bland, R. D.: Otitis Media in the First Six Weeks of Life: Diagnosis,
Bacteriology and Management. Pediatrics, 49:187, 1972.

5. P. AERUGINOSA IS MOST OFTEN ISOLATED FROM WHICH SOURCE
IN HOSPITALS?:
A. Sink trap
B. Food
C. Floor
D. Air
E. None of the above

Ref. Whitby, J. L., Rampling, A.: Pseudomonas Aeruginosa Contamination
in Domestic and Hospital Environments. Lancet, 1:15, 1972

6. WHICH OF THE FOLLOWING IS THE MOST COMMON SPECIES OF
BRUCELLA ISOLATED FROM BLOOD OF AMERICAN PATIENTS?:
A. B. abortus
B. B. suis
C. B. melitensis
D. Unknown species
E. Mixed infection

Ref. Busch, L. A., Parker, R. L.: Brucellosis in the United States.
J Infect Dis, 125:289, 1972

7.   INFECTED MULTIPLE MYELOMA PATIENTS WITH SEPSIS CAN BE
      DIFFERENTIATED FROM INFECTED MULTIPLE MYELOMA PATIENTS
      WITHOUT SEPSIS BY:
      A. Age   D. White blood cell count
      B. Serum calcium   E. None of the above
      C. BUN
      Ref. Meyers, B. R., Hirschman, S. Z., Axelrod, J. A.: Current
      Patterns of Infection in Multiple Myeloma. Amer J Med 52:87, 1972.

8.   WHICH OF THE FOLLOWING TESTS WILL MOST RAPIDLY DIFFEREN-
      TIATE SERRATIA sp FROM ENTEROBACTER sp?:
      A. Raffinose   D. Acid phosphatase production
      B. Indole   E. Citrate
      C. Motility
      Ref. Wolf, P. L., vonder Muehll, E., Ludwick, M.: A New Test to
      Differentiate Serratia from Enterobacter. Am J Clin Path, 57:241, 1972.

9.   A SIGNIFICANT NUMBER OF ENTEROBACTER SPECIES (E. AEROGENES
      E. CLOACAE, E. HAFNIA) ARE SENSITIVE TO:
      A. Penicillin   D. Carbenicillin
      B. Ampicillin   E. Cephalothin
      C. Cephaloridine
      Ref. Neu, H. C., Winshell, E. B.: Relation of B-Lactamase Activity
      and Cellular Location to Resistance of Enterobacter to Penicillins and
      Cephalosporins. Antimicrob Ag Chemother, 1:107, 1972.

10.   RITTER'S DISEASE IS PROBABLY CAUSED BY WHICH OF THE FOL-
      LOWING STAPHYLOCOCCAL TOXINS?:
      A. Alpha   D. Exfoliative toxin
      B. Beta   E. Coagulase
      C. Delta
      Ref. Melish, M. E., Glasgow, L. A., Turner, M. D.: The Staphylococcal
      Scalded-Skin Syndrome: Isolation and Partial Characterization of the
      Exfoliative Toxin. J Infect Dis, 125:129, 1972.

11.   THE MOST COMMON SALMONELLA SPECIES ISOLATED FROM
      HUMAN SOURCES IN THE UNITED STATES IN 1970 WAS:
      A. S. typhi   D. S. cholerasuis
      B. S. infantis   E. S. typhimurium
      C. S. newport
      Ref. Fox, M. D., Lowenstein, M. S., Martin, S. M.: Salmonella
      Surveillance 1970. J Infect Dis, 125:196, 1972

12.   THE BACTERIA MOST FREQUENTLY ISOLATED FROM BLOOD
      DURING SEPTIC COMPLICATIONS OF WAR WOUNDS ARE:
      A. Enterobacter group   D. Mima-Herellea
      B. Serratia marcescens   E. Enterococci
      C. Pseudomonas aeruginosa
      Ref. Tong, M. J.: Septic Complications of War Wounds. JAMA, 219:1044,
      1972.

13. IN COMPARING THE RELIABILITY OF IDENTIFICATION OF BETA
    HEMOLYTIC STREPTOCOCCI IN PRIVATE PHYSICIANS' OFFICES WITH
    REFERENCE LABORATORIES, THE PRIVATE OFFICE IS LIKELY TO:
    A. Miss 20-30% of the positive cultures
    B. Find more false-positive specimens when large numbers of strepto-
       cocci are obtained by culture
    C. Find more false-positive specimens when small numbers of strepto-
       cocci are obtained by culture
    D. Miss over 50% of the positive cultures even when confluent growth is
       present
    E. None of the above
    Ref. Battle, C. U. , Glasgow, L. A. : Reliability of Bacteriologic
    Identification of B-Hemolytic Streptococci in Private Offices. Amer J
    Dis Child, 122:134, 1971.

14. WHICH OF THE FOLLOWING IS THE MOST COMMON SIGN OF
    NEUROSYPHILIS AS SEEN IN THE LAST 10 YEARS IN THE USA?:
    A. Mania   D. Chorioretinitis
    B. Absence of tendon reflexes   E. Babinski sign
    C. Ptosis
    Ref. Hooshmand, H. , Escobar, M. , Kopf, S. W. : Neurosyphilis.
    JAMA, 219:726, 1972

15. A 23 YEAR-OLD WOMAN IN THE SECOND TRIMESTER OF HER
    SECOND PREGNANCY IS REFERRED BECAUSE OF THE FOLLOWING
    SEROLOGIC RESULTS: VDRL 1:16, FTA-ABS POSITIVE. SHE IS NOT
    ALLERGIC TO PENICILLIN. ADEQUATE TREATMENT WOULD
    INVOLVE:
    A. 600,000 u aqueous procaine penicillin injected daily for 5 days
    B. 1.2 million u aqueous procaine penicillin injected daily for 10 days;
       repeat serology monthly until delivery
    C. Tetracycline 1 gm orally per day for 30 days, repeat serology at
       end of therapy
    D. Benzathine penicillin, single injection of 4.8 million units, repeat
       serology at delivery
    E. Benzathine penicillin, 2.4 million units once per week for three weeks
    Ref. The Medical Letter, 13:85, 1971.

16. WHICH OF THE FOLLOWING IS SIGNIFICANTLY ASSOCIATED WITH THE
    RISK OF RHEUMATIC FEVER RECURRENCE AFTER STREPTOCOCCAL
    INFECTIONS?:
    A. Yearly family income
    B. Ethnic group
    C. Magnitude of rise in antistreptolysin -O titer
    D. Rheumatic fever in siblings
    E. Presence of sore throat and fever
    Ref. Spagnuolo, M. , Pasternack, B. , Taranta, A. : Risk of Rheumatic
    Fever Recurrences After Streptococcal Infections. New Eng J Med,
    285:641, 1971.

17. WHICH OF THE FOLLOWING ORGANISMS IS MOST LIKELY TO BE
    ISOLATED FROM LIVER OR LUNG WHEN POSTMORTEM CULTURES
    ARE PERFORMED, REGARDLESS OF THE CAUSE OF DEATH?:
    A. P. mirabilis   D. C. albicans
    B. S. aureus   E. Clostridium sp.
    C. E. coli
    Ref. Dolan, C. T. , Brown, A. L. , Ritts, R. E. : Microbiological
    Examination of Postmortem Tissues. Arch Path, 92:206, 1971.

18.   WHICH OF THE FOLLOWING STATEMENTS IS CORRECT CONCERNING
       STREPTOCOCCAL PHARYNGITIS IN THE GENERAL POPULATION?:
       A.   Penicillin and sulfonamide therapy are equally effective in
            eradicating streptococci from the throat
       B.   75-80% of patients with rheumatic fever give a history of sore throat
       C.   The attack rate of rheumatic fever is highest in those who have sore
            throat, Group A streptococci in the throat, and a rising ASO titer
       D.   Signs and symptoms of pharyngitis are relieved more quickly by
            penicillin than by sulfonamide therapy
       E.   Streptococcal pharyngitis can be consistently predicted from the
            clinical signs and symptoms
       Ref. Valkenburg, H. A. , Haverkorn, M. J. , Goslings, W. R. O. , et al:
       Streptococcal Pharyngitis in the General Population. J Infect Dis, 124:348,
       1971.

19.   WHICH OF THE FOLLOWING TESTS ARE NOT SPECIFIC FOR TREPO-
       NEMAL ANTIBODIES?:
       A.   Treponema pallidum immobilization (TPI)
       B.   Rapid cardiolipin test
       C.   Fluorescent treponemal antibody absorption test (FTA)
       D.   T. pallidum macrohemagglutination test
       Ref. LeClair, R. A. : Evaluation of a Qualitative Hemagglutination Test
       for Antibodies to Treponema Pallidum. J Infect Dis, 123:668, 1971.

20.   THE PRIMARY CAUSE OF FAILURE IN PREVENTING ACUTE
       RHEUMATIC FEVER FOLLOWING TREATMENT OF STREPTOCOCCAL
       PHARYNGITIS IS:
       A.   Penicillin-resistant streptococci
       B.   Inactivation of penicillin by penicillinase producing organisms
       C.   Patient failure to take drug
       D.   Persistence of the infecting streptococcus
       E.   Unusual M types of streptococci
       Ref. Catanzaro, F. J. , Rammelkamp, C. H. , Chamovitz, R. : Prevention
       of Rheumatic Fever by Treatment of Streptococcal Infections.
       New Eng J Med, 259:51, 1958.

21.   THE MOST CONSISTENT LABORATORY FINDING IN BACTEROIDES
       BACTEREMIA IS:
       A.   Anemia   D.   Hyperbilirubinemia
       B.   Hematuria   E.   Leukocytosis
       C.   Proteinuria
       Ref. Felner, J. M. , Dowell, V. R. : "Bacterioides" Bacteremia.
       Amer J Med, 50:787, 1971.

22.   MENINGITIS HAS BEEN PRODUCED IN HUMANS BY WHICH OF THE
       FOLLOWING SEROLOGIC SUBDIVISIONS OF NEISSERIA MENINGITIDIS?:
       A.   X   D.   A
       B.   Y   E.   All of the above
       C.   Z
       Ref. Fallon, R J. , Brown, W. : Infections Caused by Meningococci of
       Serogroup Z. Lancet, 1:783, 1971.

23. THE MOST LIKELY OUTCOME OF ADEQUATELY TREATED
STAPHYLOCOCCAL PNEUMONIA IN CHILDHOOD IS:
A. Recurrent respiratory tract infections
B. No residual respiratory symptoms or abnormal physical findings
C. Localized cylindrical bronchiectasis
D. Abnormal pulmonary function tests on exercise
E. Chronic bronchitis
Ref. Ceruti, E. , Contreras, J. , Neira, M. : Staphylococcal Pneumonia
in Childhood. Am J Dis Child, 122:386, 1971.

24. ELEVATIONS OF CEREBROSPINAL FLUID N-ACETYLNEURAMINIC
ACID ARE CORRELATED WITH WHICH OF THE FOLLOWING IN
REFERENCE TO BACTERIAL MENINGITIS?:
A. N. meningitidis etiology
B. H. influenza etiology
C. Recovery without neurologic sequelae
D. Coma and bacteremia
E. None of the above
Ref. O'Toole, R. D. , Goode, L. , Howe, C. : Neuraminidase Activity in
Bacterial Meningitis. J Clin Invest, 50:979, 1971.

25. THE ORGANISM MOST COMMONLY RESPONSIBLE FOR BACTEREMIA
BOTH BEFORE AND AFTER TRANSPLANTATION OF THE KIDNEY IS:
A. Bacteroides sp.   D. P. aeruginosa
B. S. viridans   E. S. pneumoniae
C. S. aureus
Ref. Leigh, D. A. : Bacteremia in Patients Receiving Human Cadaveric
Renal Transplants. J Clin Path, 24:295, 1971.

26. THE MOST COMMON NEOPLASM ASSOCIATED WITH BACTEROIDES
BACTEREMIA IS:
A. Adenocarcinoma of the colon   D. Pharyngeal carcinoma
B. Cervical or uterine tumor   E. Multiple myeloma
C. Leukemia
Ref. Felner, J. M. , Dowell, V. R. : "Bacteroides" Bacteremia.
Amer J Med, 50:787, 1971.

27. CONDITIONS NECESSARY FOR DEVELOPMENT OF INFECTION OF THE
BILIARY TRACT ARE:
A. Septicemia   D. Generally not known
B. Gallstones   E. Bile stasis
C. Bile-resistant organisms
Ref. Scott, A. J. : Bacteria and Disease of the Biliary Tract.
Gut, 12:487, 1971.

28. THE MORTALITY RATE OF NEONATAL MENINGITIS IS:
A. 5%   D. 20%
B. 65-70%   E. 30%
C. .015%
Ref. Riley, H. D. : Neonatal Meningitis. J Inf Dis, 125:420, 1972.

29. THE MOST COMMON SPECIES OF SHIGELLA ISOLATED FROM
BACILLARY DYSENTERY IN THE U. S. IS:
A. S. sonnei   D. S. boydii
B. S. dysenteriae   E. None of the above
C. S. flexneri
Ref. Lewis, J. N. , Loewenstein, M. S. : Shigellosis in the United States,
1970. J Inf Dis, 125:441, 1972.

30.   THE MOST COMMON ORGANISM CAUSING NEONATAL MENINGITIS IS:
       A. D. pneumoniae   D. E. coli
       B. Pseudomonas aeruginosa   E. S. aureus
       C. Proteus sp.
       Ref. Bush, R. T.: Purulent Meningitis of the Newborn: A Survey of 28
       Cases. New Zealand Med J, 73:278, 1971.

31.   THE MOST NEARLY CORRECT NUMBER FOR CASES OF GONORRHEA
       PER 100,000 IN THE UNITED STATES IN 1970 WAS:
       A. 285   D. 2,000
       B. 130   E. 730
       C. 5
       Ref. Lucas, J. B.: Gonococcal Resistance to Antibiotics. South Med Bull,
       59:22, 1971.

32.   AN OPERATING ROOM IS TO BE FITTED WITH ULTRAVIOLET LIGHT
       FIXTURES FOR AIR DISINFECTION. IN REFERENCE TO AIR
       CIRCULATION:
       A. Cold air should enter the bottom of the room
       B. Hot air should enter the bottom of the room
       C. Cold air should enter the top of the room
       D. Hot air should enter the top of the room
       Ref. Riley, R. L., Permutt, S., Kaufman, J. E.: Room Air Disinfection
       by Ultraviolet Irradiation of Upper Air. Arch Environ Health,
       23:35, 1971.

33.   THE MAJOR CHANGE IN TRACHEOBRONCHIAL SECRETIONS
       DURING TRACHEOBRONCHIAL INFECTION IS:
       A. Increase in lysozyme concentration
       B. Appearance of IgM
       C. Decrease in lactoferrin concentration
       D. Increase in volume of secretions
       E. Decrease in sialomucin concentration
       Ref. Yeager, H., Jr.: Tracheobronchial Secretions. Amer J Med,
       50:493, 1971.

34.   WHICH OF THE FOLLOWING SUBSTANCES USED IN PROCESSING
       BLOOD CULTURES SHOULD YOU SUSPECT AFTER A NUMBER OF
       FALSE POSITIVE BLOOD CULTURES HAVE APPEARED IN YOUR
       LABORATORY?:
       A. Thioglycollate broth   D. Thiol broth
       B. Penicillinase   E. Prepackaged pipettes
       C. Sodium citrate
       Ref. Faris, H. M., Sparling, F. D.: Mima Polymorpha Bacteremia.
       JAMA, 219:76, 1972.

35.   LISTED BELOW ARE SEVERAL SYSTEMS FOR PERFORMING
       ANAEROBIC BACTERIAL CULTURES. SELECT THE SIMPLEST
       AND ALSO THE MOST EFFECTIVE SYSTEM:
       A. Anaerobically sterilized plated media pre-reduced
       B. The roll tube method using pre-reduced media
       C. Self-contained anaerobic models
       D. Gaspack[R] system
       E. Replacement of air with hydrogen and CO_2
       Ref. Rosenblatt, J. E., Fallon, A. M., Finegold, S. M.: Comparison
       of Culture Methods for Isolation of Anaerobes from Clinical Specimens.
       Clin Res, 20:189, 1972.

36. NOSOCOMIAL INFECTIONS ARE MOST COMMON ON WHICH SERVICE IN MOST HOSPITALS GIVING CARE TO ACUTELY ILL PATIENTS?:
    A. Medicine
    B. Surgery
    C. Pediatrics
    D. Gynecology
    E. Obstetrics
    Ref. Sencer, D. J.: Emerging Diseases of Man and Animals. Ann Rev Microbiol, 25:465, 1971.

37. A POSTMORTEM BLOOD CULTURE CONTAINING ANAEROBIC BACTERIA IS MOST LIKELY TO HAVE BEEN ASSOCIATED WITH WHICH OF THE FOLLOWING ANTE-MORTEM CONDITIONS?:
    A. Peritonitis
    B. Bowel hemorrhage
    C. Mesenteric thrombosis
    D. Ulcerative bowel lesions
    E. All of the above
    Ref. Kuklinca, A. G., Gavan, T. L.: Anaerobic Bacteria in Postmortem Blood Cultures. Cleveland Clin Quart, 38:5, 1971.

38. AN INFANT OR CHILD WITH ACUTE APPENDICITIS WITH PERFOR-ATION WOULD BE MOST LIKELY TO DEVELOP WHICH OF THE FOL-LOWING COMPLICATIONS?:
    A. Acute orchitis
    B. Wound abscess
    C. Intestinal obstruction
    D. Fecal fistula
    E. Gram negative bacillary sepsis
    Ref. Holgersen, L. O., Stanley-Brown, E. G.: Acute Appendicitis with Perforation. Amer J Dis Child, 122:288, 1971.

39. WHICH OF THE FOLLOWING COMBINATIONS OF SIGNS AND SYMPTOMS WOULD BE MOST COMPATIBLE WITH APPENDICITIS AND PERFORATION IN AN INFANT OR CHILD?:
    A. Abdominal pain in the right lower abdomen, nausea-vomiting, fever
    B. Diarrhea, anorexia, constipation
    C. Abdominal mass, abdominal distention, fever
    D. Decreased bowel sounds, constipation, fever
    E. Rigid abdomen, mass by rectal exam, abdominal pain
    Ref. Holgersen, L. O., Stanley-Brown, E. G.: Acute Appendicitis with Perforation. Amer J Dis Child, 122:288, 1971.

40. SPLIT THICKNESS SKIN GRAFTS WHEN TESTED IN VITRO AS DISCS ON AN AGAR PLATE SHOW ANTIBACTERIAL ACTIVITY AGAINST:
    A. P. aeruginosa
    B. E. coli
    C. S. aureus
    D. All the organisms above
    E. None of the organisms above
    Ref. Rubin, L. R., Bongiovi, J., Jr.: Human Skin-Antibacterial In Vitro? J Surg Res, 11:321, 1971.

41. MOST INFECTIONS ACQUIRED IN A COMMUNITY TEACHING HOSPITAL WITH A GENERAL MEDICAL POPULATION COME FROM:
    A. Urinary catheters
    B. Inhalation therapy
    C. Cardiac catheterizations
    D. Intravenous catheterization
    E. Surgical wounds
    Ref. Groschel, D., Bradley, S. R.: Surveillance of Infections in a Community Teaching Hospital. Yale J Biol Med, 44:247, 1971.

42.   WHICH OF THE FOLLOWING IS MOST EFFECTIVE IN REDUCING THE
       NUMBER OF DAYS FEBRILE AFTER SURGERY FOR RUPTURED
       APPENDIX?:
       A. Topical antibiotics to the wound
       B. Intraoperative intraperitoneal antibiotics
       C. Systemic antibiotic therapy
       D. Peritoneal drainage
       E. Both C and D above
       Ref. Margarey, C. J., Chant, A. D. B., Rickford, C. R. K., et al:
       Peritoneal Drainage and Systemic Antibiotics After Appendicitis. Lancet,
       24 July 1971, p. 179

43.   RESISTANCE TO RIFAMYCIN AMONG GRAM-NEGATIVE BACILLI IS
       PROBABLY BY WHICH OF THE FOLLOWING MECHANISMS?:
       A. Cell becomes impermeable to rifampin
       B. Cell destroys rifampin
       C. RNA polymerase develops which does not complex with rifampin
       D. Rifampin binds to extracts of mutant cells
       E. None of the above
       Ref. Wehrli, W., Staehlin, M.: Action of the Rifamycins. Bact Rev,
       35:290, 1971.

44.   THE MOST COMMON ANAEROBIC ORGANISM ISOLATED IN MIXED
       CULTURE FROM WOUNDS WHICH CONTAIN ANAEROBIC GRAM-
       POSITIVE COCCI IS:
       A. Catenabacterium   D. Clostridium
       B. Bacteroides   E. Bifidobacterium
       C. Fusobacterium
       Ref. Pien, F. D., Thompson, R. L., Martin, W. J.: Clinical and
       Bacteriologic Studies of Anaerobic Gram-Positive Cocci. Mayo Clin Proc,
       47:251, 1972.

45.   THE MOST COMMON AEROBIC ORGANISM ISOLATED IN MIXED
       CULTURE FROM WOUNDS WHICH CONTAIN ANAEROBIC GRAM-
       POSITIVE COCCI IS:
       A. Staphylococci   D. Bacteroides
       B. Candida   E. Pseudomonas
       C. Proteus
       Ref. Pien, F. D., Thompson, R. L., Martin, W. J.: Clinical and
       Bacteriologic Studies of Anaerobic Gram-Positive Cocci. Mayo Clin Proc,
       47:251, 1972.

46.   THE PRODUCT OF S. AUREUS THOUGHT TO BE RESPONSIBLE FOR THE
       SCALDED SKIN SYNDROME IS:
       A. Alpha toxin   D. Exfoliatin
       B. Delta toxin   E. Beta hemolysin
       C. Coagulase
       Ref. Kapral, F. A., Miller, M. M.: Product of Staphylococcus Aureus
       Responsible for the Scalded Skin Syndrome. Inf and Imm, 4:541, 1971.

47.   SALMONELLA MENINGITIS OF NEWBORNS IS CHARACTERIZED BY ALL
       OF THE FOLLOWING, EXCEPT:
       A. Rapid clinical course
       B. Low mortality rate
       C. Preceding diarrhea
       D. Epidemic outbreak
       E. Negative Kernig and Brudzinski sign
       Ref. Rabinowitz, S. G., MacLeod, N. R.: Salmonella Meningitis.
       Amer J Dis Child, 123:259, 1972.

48. THE MOST COMMON ORGANISM RESPONSIBLE FOR OSTEOMYELITIS
     OF THE HIP IS:
     A. E. coli   D. S. aureus
     B. P. aeruginosa   E. S. pyogenes
     C. S. cholerasuis
     Ref. Waldvogel, F. A. , Medoff, G. , Swartz, M. N. : Osteomyelitis.
     N Eng J Med, 282:260, 1970.

49. ASSUMING THAT NO GALLBLADDER DISEASE IS PRESENT, WHAT
     PERCENTAGE OF CHRONIC CARRIERS OF TYPHOID BACILLI WILL
     BE CURED AFTER TAKING 4-6 gm OF AMPICILLIN ORALLY FOR AT
     LEAST 28 DAYS?:
     A. 10%   D. 70%
     B. 40%   E. 25%
     C. 99%
     Ref. Phillips, W. E. : Treatment of Chronic Typhoid Carriers with
     Ampicillin. JAMA, 217:913, 1971.

50. WHICH OF THE FOLLOWING IS OF LEAST VALUE IN ESTABLISHING
     THE DIAGNOSIS OF PNEUMOCOCCAL PNEUMONIA?:
     A. Clinical diagnosis
     B. Examination of Gram's stain of sputum
     C. Culture of trans-tracheal aspirate
     D. Culture of sputum
     E. Blood culture
     Ref. Barrett-Connor, E. : Non-value of Sputum Culture in the Diagnosis
     of Pneumococcal Pneumonia. Amer Rev Resp Dis, 103:845, 1971.

51. WHICH OF THE FOLLOWING MOST RELIABLY SEPARATES
     S. AUREUS FROM S. EPIDERMIDIS?:
     A. Sheep blood hemolysin
     B. Pigment production
     C. Colonial morphology
     D. Catalase production
     E. Coagulase production
     Ref. Gunn, B. A. , Dunkelberg, W. E. , Creitz, J. R. : Clinical Evaluation
     of 2% - LSM Medium for Primary Isolation and Identification of
     Staphylococci. Amer J Clin Path, 57:237, 1972.

52. THE MICROSCOPIC FEATURES OF THE SKIN LESION OF PSEUDOMONAS
     SEPSIS INCLUDE:
     A. Invasion of vein wall by bacteria
     B. Little accompanying inflammatory exudate
     C. Intimal involvement
     D. Early necrosis of small arteries
     Ref. Dorff, G. J. , Geimer, N. F. , Rosenthal, D. R. , et al: Pseudomonas
     Septicemia. Arch Intern Med, 128:591, 1971.

53. PATIENTS INFECTED WITH PASTEURELLA PSEUDOTUBERCULOSIS
     ARE MOST LIKELY TO HAVE DYSFUNCTION OF WHICH OF THE
     FOLLOWING ORGANS?:
     A. Lung   D. Heart
     B. Brain   E. Liver
     C. Bowel
     Ref. Yamashiro, K. , Goldman, R. H. , Harris, D. : Pasturella
     Pseudotuberculosis. Arch Intern Med, 128:605, 1971.

54. THE FOLLOWING ARE CAUSES OF CREPITANT NONCLOSTRIDIAL
CELLULITIS:
A. Infection with bacteroides organisms
B. Anaerobic streptococcal infection
C. Coliform infections
D. Hemolytic streptococcal infection
E. All of the above
Ref. Altemeier, W. A., Fullen, W. D.,: Prevention and Treatment of
Gas Gangrene. JAMA, 217:806, 1971.

55. COMPARING ROUTINE MEDIA FOR IDENTIFICATION OF ENTERIC
BACTERIA WITH ENTEROTUBES (SINGLE TUBE CONTAINING EIGHT
CULTURE MEDIA IN SEPARATE COMPARTMENTS), DISAGREEMENT
IS MOST OFTEN ENCOUNTERED IN IDENTIFYING:
A. E. coli   D. Klebsiella sp.
B. P. mirabilis   E. Salmonella sp.
C. Pseudomonas aeruginosa
Ref. Morton, H. E., Monaco, M. A. J.: Comparison of Enterotubes and
Routine Media for the Identification of Enteric Bacteria. Amer J Clin
Pathol, 56:64, 1971.

56. THE ORGANISM CULTURED MOST FREQUENTLY FROM AREAS OF
"DIAPER" DERMATITIS IS:
A. G. tetragena
B. S. aureus
C. E. coli
D. Corynebacterium species
E. C. albicans
Ref. Montes, L. F., Dittillo, R. F., Hunt, D., et al: Microbial Flora
of Infants' Skin. Arch Derm, 103:400, 1971.

THE FOLLOWING QUESTIONS CONSIST OF PAIRS OF PHRASES
DESCRIBING CONDITIONS OR QUANTITIES WHICH MAY OR MAY NOT
VARY IN RELATION TO EACH OTHER. ANSWER:
A. If increase in the first is accompanied by increase in the second or
   decrease in the first is accompanied by decrease in the second
B. If increase in the first is accompanied by decrease in the second or
   decrease in the first is accompanied by increase in the second
C. If changes in the first are independent of changes in the second

57. 1. Length of storage of platelet-rich plasma at 25°C
    2. Frequency of bacterial recovery from platelet-rich plasma stored
       at 25°C
Ref. Buchholz, D. H., Young, V. M., Friedman, N., etal: Bacterial
Proliferation in Platelet Products Stored at Room Temperature.
N Eng J Med, 285:429, 1971.

58. 1. Duration of bacteruria
    2. Urinary concentrating ability
Ref. Ronald, A. R., Cutler, R. E., Turck, M.: Effect of Bacteruria on
Renal Concentrating Mechanisms. Ann Intern Med, 70:723, 1969.

THE FOLLOWING QUESTIONS CONSIST OF A STATEMENT AND A REASON. SELECT:
A. If both statement and reason are true <u>and</u> the reason is a correct explanation of the statement
B. If both statement and reason are true <u>but</u> the reason is not a correct explanation of the statement
C. If the statement is true but the reason is false
D. If the statement is false but the reason is true
E. If both statement and reason are false

59. ____ Patients with bacterial endocarditis, aortic insufficiency, and severe heart failure should have an aortic valvular prosthesis installed as soon as possible BECAUSE patients with bacterial endocarditis, aortic insufficiency, and severe heart failure may die suddenly of embolic myocardial infarction.
Ref. Griffin, F.M., Jones, G. Cobbs, C.G.: Aortic Insufficiency in Bacterial Endocarditis. Ann Int Med, 76:23, 1972.

60. ____ Closing and cleaning of wards reduces sepsis rates and ends outbreaks of infection BECAUSE closing and cleaning a ward causes a reduction in the numbers of infections caused by both Gram negative positive and Gram negative bacteria.
Ref. Noone, P., Griffiths, R.J.: The Effect on Sepsis Rates of Closing and Cleaning Hospital Wards. J Clin Path, 24: 721 1971.

61. ____ Detection of bacteria by microscopic examination of gram-stained uncentrifuged correctly collected mid-stream urine sample is not an indication of urinary tract infection BECAUSE detection of bacteria in such a sample is not highly correlated with the presence of bacterial colony counts of greater than 10^5/ml in that urine.
Ref. Lang, G.R., Levin, S.: Diagnosis and Treatment of Urinary Tract Infections. Med Clin N Amer, 55:1439, 1971.

62. ____ The fluorescent treponemal antibody absorption test (FTA-ABS) cannot be used to evaluate effectiveness of therapy for syphilis BECAUSE the FTA-ABS test may remain positive for many years after adequate treatment for syphilis.
Ref. The Medical Letter, 13:85, 1971.

63. ____ Even though presence of syphilis is not yet established, contacts of infective syphilis should be treated for syphilis if seen within 30 days of contact BECAUSE it has been repeatedly demonstrated that, if not treated, these contacts may later be the source of a new train of infection.
Ref. Brown, W.J.: Status and Control of Syphilis in the United States. J Inf Dis, 124:428, 1971.

64. ____ Blood cultures should be obtained at regular intervals in the post treatment period for Streptococcus viridans endocarditis BECAUSE bacteriologic evidence of relapse of S. viridans endocarditis is likely to antedate subjective or objective clinical evidence.
Ref. Tan, J.S., Terhune, C.A., Jr., Kaplan, S., Hamburger, M.: Successful Two-Week Treatment Schedule for Penicillin-Susceptible Streptococcus Viridans Endocarditis. Lancet, 2:1340, 1971.

65. ____ Prevention of H. influenza meningitis should be the aim of therapy BECAUSE only about 10% of children who survive H. influenza meningitis have any neurologic deficit whatsoever.
Ref. Sell, S.H.W., Merrill, R.E., Doyne, E.O., et al: Long Term Sequalae of Hemophilus Influenzae Meningitis. Pediat, 49:206, 1972.

66. ___ The passive bacterial hemagglutination test for serum antibody may establish the diagnosis of salmonella enteritis when cultural results are negative BECAUSE serum antibody detectable by the passive bacterial hemagglutination test may achieve diagnostic titers within 48 to 72 hours after symptoms begin.
Ref. Neter, E : The Immune Response of the Host: An Aid to Etiology, Pathogenesis, Diagnosis and Epidemiology of Bacterial Infection. Yale J Biol Med, 44:241, 1971.

67. ___ If a patient has ever had Streptococcus viridans endocarditis, all teeth should be extracted BECAUSE Streptococcus viridans endocarditis has not been reported in the edentulous patient.
Ref. Simon, D. S., Goodwin, J. F.: Should Good Teeth be Extracted to Prevent Streptococcus Viridans Endocarditis? Lancet, 1:1207, 1971.

68. ___ An erythrocyte sedimentation rate of less than 40 mm/hr is compatible with osteomyelitis of the newborn BECAUSE children less than 1 month of age seldom develop an ESR greater than 40 mm/hr even when osteomyelitis is present.
Ref. Ek, J.: Acute Hematogenous Osteomyelitis in Infancy and Childhood. Clin Ped, 10:377, 1971.

69. ___ Rifampin is effective in reducing rates of meningococcal carriage by as much as 95% BECAUSE rifampin-resistant meningococcal strains do not arise after treatment.
Ref. Beam, W. E., Newberg, N. R., Devine, L. F., Pierce, W. E., Davies, J. A.: The Effect of Rifampin on the Nasopharyngeal Carriage Rate of Neisseria Meningitidis in a Military Population. J Infect Dis, 124:39, 1971.

70. ___ Anaerobic nonsporulating bacilli, which account for 99% of the total intestinal flora, persist in the bowel after use of antibiotics for preoperative bowel "sterilization" BECAUSE these bacilli are resistant to the antibiotics most often used for bowel "sterilization."
Ref. Felner, J., Dowell, V. R.: Bacteroides Bacteremia. Amer J Med, 50:787, 1971.

71. ___ A search for both otic and pulmonary foci is important in managing pneumococcal meningitis BECAUSE pneumococcal meningitis associated with a pneumonic focus is more likely to lead to death than pneumococcal meningitis from an otic focus.
Ref. Richter, R. W., Brust, J. C. M.: Pneumococcal Meningitis at Harlem Hospital. NY State J Med, 71:2747, 1971.

72. ___ Acquired stenosis of the mitral valve may occur following bacterial endocarditis BECAUSE bacterial vegetations can obstruct the lumen of the mitral valve.
Ref. Benisch, B. M.: Mitral Stenosis and Insufficiency: A Complication of Healed Bacterial Endocarditis. Am Heart J, 82:39, 1971.

73. ___ Vibrio cholerae will most probably be correctly identified by most general hospital laboratories in the United States BECAUSE the media ordinarily used to isolate enteric pathogens are also the preferred media for isolation of V. cholerae.
Ref. Balows, A., Hermann, G. J., DeWitt, W. E.: The Isolation and Identification of Vibrio Cholerae - A Review. Health Lab Sci, 8:167, 1971.

ANSWER THE FOLLOWING QUESTIONS ACCORDING TO THE KEY
BELOW:
A. If choice A is greater than choice B
B. If choice B is greater than choice A
C. If A and B are equal or nearly equal

74. RESISTANCE TO CYTOSINE ARABINOSIDE AND 6-MP OF:
     A. Pseudomonas
     B. E. coli
     Ref. Goldschmidt, M. C., Bodey, G. P.: Effect of Chemotherapeutic
     Agents Upon Microorganisms Isolated From Cancer Patients.
     Antimicrob Ag Chemother, 1:348, 1972.

75. PERCENT OF STRAINS OF PROTEUS sp, E COLI, PSEUDOMONAS,
     ENTEROBACTER RESISTANT TO:
     A. Gentamicin
     B. Tobramycin
     Ref. Del Bene, V. E., Farrar, W. E., Jr.: Tobramycin: In Vitro
     Activity and Comparison with Kanamycin and Gentamicin. Antimicrob
     Ag Chemother, 1:340, 1972.

76. RISK OF PERSISTENT CARRIAGE OF STREPTOCOCCI IN THE
     NASOPHARYNX OF:
     A. Tonsillectomized children
     B. Normal siblings
     Ref. Matonoski, G. M.: The Role of the Tonsils in Streptococcal
     Infections: A Comparison of Tonsillectomized Children and Sibling
     Controls. Amer J Epidemiol, 95:278, 1972.

77. SEROLOGICALLY AND BACTERIOLOGICALLY PROVEN STREPTO-
     COCCAL INFECTIONS OCCURRING IN AGE-MATCHED CHILDREN:
     A. After tonsillectomy
     B. Without tonsillectomy
     Ref. Matonoski, G. M.: The Role of the Tonsils in Streptococcal
     Infections: A Comparison of Tonsillectomized Children and Sibling
     Controls. Amer J Epidemiol, 95:278, 1972.

78. THE MIC OF CARBENICILLIN IN mcg/ml AGAINST:
     A. Penicillin-sensitive S. aureus
     B. Penicillinase-producing S. aureus
     Ref. Gram Negative Sepsis: Sanford, J. P., (ed). Med Com, New York,
     N. Y., 1971, p. 74

79. ACTIVITY OF:
     A. Trimethoprim against classical V. cholera
     B. Trimethoprim-sulfamethoxazole against V. cholera
     Ref. Northrup, R. S., Doyle, M. A., Feeley, J. C.: In Vitro Susceptibility
     of El Tor and Classical Vibrio Cholera Strains to Trimethoprim and
     Sulfamethoxazole. Antimicrob Ag Chemother, 1:310, 1972.

80. CURE RATES FOR GONORRHEA IN WOMEN RECEIVING:
     A. 2 gm spectinomycin
     B. 4 gm spectinomycin
     Ref. Duncan, W. C., Holder, W. R., Roberts, D. P., et al: Treatment
     of Gonorrhea with Spectinomycin Hydrochloride: Comparison with
     Standard Penicillin Schedules. Antimicrob Ag Chemother, 1:210, 1971.

81.   IN VITRO ACTIVITY OF THE FOLLOWING ANTIBIOTICS AGAINST
       SERRATIA MARCESCENS:
       A. Tobramycin
       B. Gentamicin
       Ref. Traub, W. H. , Raymond, E. A. : Evaluation of the In Vitro Activity
       of Tobramycin as Compared with that of Gentamicin Sulfate. Appl
       Microbiol, 23:4, 1972.

82.   IN REFERENCE TO COLIFORM BACILLI CAUSING URINARY TRACT
       INFECTION, RESISTANCE TO SULFONAMIDES IS MORE FREQUENTLY
       ENCOUNTERED WHEN THE INFECTION IS ACQUIRED:
       A. Outside the hospital
       B. Inside the hospital
       Ref. Gillispie, W. A. , Lee, P. A. , Linton, K. B. , et al: Antibiotic
       Resistance of Coliform Bacilli in Urinary Infection Acquired by Women
       Outside Hospital. Lancet, 2:675, 1971.

83.   INCIDENCE OF INFECTIOUS COMPLICATIONS AFFECTING A
       HOSPITALIZED PEDIATRIC POPULATION TREATED WITH:
       A. Scalp vein needles for intravenous infusion
       B. Polyethylene catheters for intravenous infusion
       Ref. Peter, G. , Lloyd-Still, J. D. , Lovejoy, F. : Local Infection and
       Bacteremia from Scalp Vein Needles and Polyethylene Catheters in
       Children. J Pediat, 80:78, 1972.

84.   THE PERCENTAGE OF STRAINS OF THE FOLLOWING ORGANISMS
       WHICH ARE RESISTANT IN VITRO TO SULFAMETHOXAZOLE-
       TRIMETHOPRIM COMBINATION:
       A. Staphylococcus
       B. Enterococcus
       Ref. Lebek, G. , Wiedmer, E. E. : In Vitro Sensitivity of Human
       Pathogens to the Combined Preparation Sulfamethoxazole-Trimethoprim.
       Schweiz Med Wochenschr, 101:1385, 1971.

85.   SERUM ALBUMIN OF:
       A   Normal rats
       B. Rats inoculated intravenously with D. pneumoniae
       Ref. Mitruka, B. M. : Biochemical Aspects of Diplococcus Pneumoniae
       Infections in Laboratory Rats. Yale J Biol Med, 44:253, 1971.

86.   INCIDENCE OF STAPHYLOCOCCAL DISEASE OF THE NEWBORN AMONG
       CHILDREN BORN TO MOTHERS IMMUNIZED BEFORE DELIVERY WITH:
       A. Monovalent capsular polysaccharide antigen from S. aureus
       B. Killed virus polymyelitis vaccine (as a control)
       Ref. Lavoipierre, G. J. , Newell, K. W. , Smith, M. H. D. , et al: A
       Vaccine Trial for Neonatal Staphylococcal Disease. Amer J Dis Child,
       122:377, 1971.

87.   GROWTH OF T-MYCOPLASMAS FROM HUMAN SOURCES ON PPLO
       MEDIA CONTAINING:
       A. Serum 20%
       B. Serum (20%) plus .05% thallium acetate
       Ref. Lee, Y. H. , Bailey, P. E. , McCormack, W. M. : T-Mycoplasma
       from Urine and Vaginal Specimens: Decreased Rates of Isolation and
       Growth in the Presence of Thallium Acetate. J Infec Dis, 125:318, 1972.

88.   BACTERICIDAL EFFECTIVENESS OF KANAMYCIN AGAINST:
       A. S. aureus
       B. D. pneumoniae
       Ref. Bunn, P. A. : Kanamycin. Med Clin N Amer, 54:1245, 1970.

89. SUSCEPTIBILITY OF M. PNEUMONIAE IN VITRO TO:
   A. Erythromycin
   B. Tetracycline
   Ref. Jao, R. L. , Finland, M. : Susceptibility of M. Pneumoniae to 21
   Antibiotics In Vitro. Amer J Med Sci, 253:639, 1967.

90. NUMBER OF STRAINS OF MENINGOCOCCI RESISTANT TO RIFAMPIN
   WHICH ARE PRESENT IN A:
   A. Small inoculum
   B. Large inoculum
   Ref. O'Bierne, A. , Robinson, J. A. : Sensitivity of Neiserria Meningitidis
   to Rifampin, Penicillin, and Sulfadiazine. Amer J Med Sci, 262:33, 1971.

91. PERCENTAGE OF SALMONELLA TYPHIMURIUM STRAINS RESISTANT TO:
   A. Streptomycin
   B. Tetracycline
   Ref. Cherubin, C. E. , Szmuness, M. , Winter, J. : Antibiotic Resistance
   of Salmonella. NY State J Med, 72:369, 1972.

92. APPEARANCE OF PROTEUS sp. NOSOCOMIAL INFECTIONS:
   A. On surgical wards
   B. In medical wards
   Ref. Adler, J. , Burke, J. P. , Martin, D. F. , Finland, M. : Proteus
   Infections in a General Hospital; II: Some Clinical and Epidemiological
   Characteristics. Ann Intern Med, 75:531-536, 1971.

93. INCIDENCE OF PULMONARY INFECTIONS AFTER:
   A. Renal transplantation
   B. Cardiac transplantation
   Ref. Gurwurth, M. J. , Stinson, E. B. , Remington, J. S. : Aspergillus
   Infection Complicating Cardiac Transplantation. Arch Int Med, 128:541,
   1971.

94. INCIDENCE OF:
   A. Neurologic sequelae following meningococcal meningitis
   B. Hypotension during meningococcal meningitis
   Ref. Everett, E. D. : Complications and Residuals of Meningococcal
   Disease. Military Medicine, 136:612, 1971.

95. PERCENT OF PATIENTS WITH CHRONIC BRONCHITIS WHO HAVE
   SERUM BACTERICIDAL ANTIBODY AGAINST:
   A. H. influenzae, Type B
   B. H. Influenzae, unencapsulated
   Ref. Gump, D. W. , Tarr, P. , Philipps, A. , et al: Bactericidal
   Antibodies to Hemophilus Influenzae. Proc Soc Exp Biol Med, 138:76,
   1971.

96. INCIDENCE OF GONOCOCCAL ARTHRITIS IN:
   A. Men
   B. Women
   Ref. Ellner, P. D. : Diagnosis of Gonococcal Infection. Clin Med, 78:16,
   1971.

97. NUMBER OF VIABLE:
   A. S. typhi cells which must be ingested to produce disease
   B. S. flexneri cells which must be ingested to produce disease
   Ref. DuPont, H. L. , Hornick, R. B. , Snyder, M. J. , et al: Immunity in
   Shigellosis II Protection Induced by Oral Live Vaccine or Primary
   Infection. J Inf Dis, 125:12, 1972.

98.   FREQUENCY OF GRAM NEGATIVE BACTEREMIA AMONG PATIENTS
      HOSPITALIZED ON:
      A. Burn units
      B. Cardiac surgery recovery units
      Ref. Sanford, J. P. , Fekety, F. R. , Jr. , Geddes, A. M. , Ohkoshi, M. ,
      Turck, M. : Panel Discussion of the Treatment of Serious Gram
      Negative Infections. Postgrad Med J, Feb. 1971 supplement, pp. 135-142

99.   FATALITIES DUE TO GRAM NEGATIVE BACILLEMIA AMONG
      PATIENTS WITH:
      A. Carcinoma
      B. Leukemia
      Ref. Myerowitz, R. L. , Medeiros, A. A. , O'Brien, T. F. : Recent
      Experience with Bacillemia due to Gram-Negative Organisms.
      J Inf Dis, 124:239, 1971.

100. PERCENTAGE OF PATIENTS WITH LATE LATENT SYPHILIS WHOSE
      SERUM WILL GIVE A POSITIVE:
      A. Fluorescent treponemal antibody absorption test
      B. Wasserman test
      Ref. Foster, M. T. : Diagnosis and Treatment of Venereal Disease.
      Posgrad Med, 50:66, 1971.

101. CHANCE THAT PARTIAL ANTIBIOTIC THERAPY WILL:
      A. Sterilize cerebrospinal fluid in meningococcal meningitis
      B. Alter leukocyte count, protein and glucose content toward normal in
          meningococcal meningitis
      Ref. Dalton, H. P. , Allison, M. J. : Modification of Laboratory Results
      by Partial Treatment of Bacterial Meningitis. Amer J Clin Path,
      49:410, 1968.

102. THE MEDIAN MIC (MICROGRAMS/ML) AGAINST E. COLI OF:
      A. Penicillin G
      B. Methicillin
      Ref. Gilbert, D. N. , Sanford, J. P. : Methicillin: Critical Appraisal
      After a Decade of Experience. Med Clin N Amer, 54:1113, 1970.

103. THE MEDIAN MIC (MICROGRAMS/ML) AGAINST N. MENINGITIDIS OF:
      A. Phenoxymethylpenicillin
      B. Benzylpenicillin
      Ref. Sabath, L. D. : Phenoxymethylpenicillin (Penicillin V) and
      Phenethicillin. Med Clin N Amer, 54:1101, 1970.

104. MEAN AGE OF PATIENTS WITH ENDOCARDITIS IN:
      A. 1938
      B. 1966
      Ref. Cherubin, C. E. , Neu, H. C. : Infective Endocarditis at the
      Presbyterian Hospital in New York City from 1938-1967. Amer J Med,
      51:83, 1971.

EACH SET OF LETTERED HEADINGS IS FOLLOWED BY A NUMBERED
LIST OF WORDS OR PHRASES. ANSWER:
A. If the word or phrase is associated with A only
B. If the word or phrase is associated with B only
C. If the word or phrase is associated with both A and B
D. If the word or phrase is associated with neither A nor B

A. Pasturella multocida
B. Yersinia pseudotuberculosis
C. Both
D. Neither

105. ___ Dog bite
106. ___ Mesenteric adenitis
107. ___ Cat bite
108. ___ Superficial leg ulcers
Ref. Pasturella and Yersinia Infections - United Kingdom Morb. Mort
Weekly Rep, 21:146, 1972.

A. Motile
B. Oxidase positive
C. Both
D. Neither

109. ___ Bordetella bronchoseptica
110. ___ Alcaligenes species
111. ___ Pseudomonas maltophilia
112. ___ Pseudomonas aeruginosa
113. ___ Mima polymorpha
114. ___ Herellea vaginicola
Ref. Gardner, P. , Griffin, W. B. , Swartz, M. N. , et al: Nonfermentative
Gram-Negative Bacilli of Nosocomial Interest. Amer J Med, 48:735, 1970.

A. Bordetella bronchiseptica
B. Brucella melitensis
C. Both
D. Neither

115. ___ CO_2 requirement
116. ___ Urease positive
117. ___ Utilize citrate
118. ___ Oxidase positive
119. ___ Growth on MacConkeys agar
Ref. Swenson, R. M. , Carmichael, L. E. , Cundy, K. R. : Human Infection
with Brucella Canis. Ann Int Med, 76:435, 1972.

A.   Bacterial endocarditis
B.   Systemic lupus erythematosus
C.   Both
D.   Neither

120. ___ May be associated with nephritis
121. ___ Hypocomplementemia
122. ___ Elevated titers of anti-gamma globulin
123. ___ Sudden onset of aortic valvular insufficiency
124. ___ Anti-DNA anti-nuclear antibodies most common
125. ___ Negative blood cultures
Ref. Gutman, R. A., Striker, G. E., Gilliland, B. C., et al: The Immune
Complex Glomerulonephritis of Bacterial Endocarditis. Medicine,
51:1, 1972.

A.   Renal bacteruria
B.   Bladder bacteruria
C.   Both
D.   Neither

126. ___ Frequency of urination
127. ___ Burning on urination
128. ___ Suprapubic pain
129. ___ Rigors
130. ___ Hematuria
131. ___ Loin pain
Ref. Fairley, K. F., Carson, N. E., Gutch, R. C., et al: Site of Infection
in Acute Urinary Tract Infection in General Practice. Lancet, 2:615,
1971.

A.   Rocky Mountain spotted fever
B.   Rickettsialpox
C.   Both
D.   Neither

132. ___ Tick bite
133. ___ Mite bite
134. ___ Eschar
135. ___ Rodent reservoir
136. ___ Negative Weil - Felix reaction
Ref. Murray, E. S.: Rickettsial Diseases in Textbook of Medicine.
Beeson, P. B., McDermott, W., (ed), W. B. Saunders Co., Philadelphia,
1971, p. 470.

A. Pseudomonas aeruginosa
B. Pseudomonas pseudomallei
C. Both
D. Neither

137. ___ Gram negative
138. ___ Acid fast
139. ___ Sporebearing
140. ___ Hemolytic
141. ___ Motile
142. ___ Oxidase positive
143. ___ No soluble pigment production
144. ___ Growth at 42°C

Ref. Howe, C., Sampath, A., Spotnitz, M.: The Pseudomallei Group: A Review. J Inf Dis, 124:598, 1972.

A. Bacterial endocarditis
B. Fungal endocarditis
C. Both
D. Neither

145. ___ Positive blood cultures infrequent
146. ___ Focal glomerular lesions
147. ___ Major arterial embolization
148. ___ Chemotherapy usually successful

Ref. Drutz, D.J.: The Spectrum of Fungal Endocarditis. Calif Med, 115:34, 1971.

A. Staphylococcus
B. Streptococcus
C. Both
D. Neither

149. ___ Paronychia
150. ___ Terminal pulp infection
151. ___ Acute cellulitis of the hand
152. ___ Tendon sheath infection
153. ___ Infective arthritis
154. ___ Erysipeloid

Ref. Sneddon, J.: The Care of Hand Infections. Baltimore. The Williams and Wilkins Co., 1970.

A. Vesicle
B. Papule
C. Both
D. Neither

155. ___ Anthrax
156. ___ Catscratch fever
157. ___ Diphtheria
158. ___ Granuloma inguinale
159. ___ Primary syphilis
160. ___ Herpes zoster
161. ___ Rocky Mountain spotted fever
162. ___ Chicken pox

Ref. Fekerty, F.R., Cluff, L.E.: The Clinical and Laboratory Manifestations of Infectious Diseases in The Principles and Practice of Medicine, 17th Ed, Chap 6, Appleton-Century-Crofts, New York, 1968, pp. 654-671.

A.   Bacteroides bacteremia
B.   Fusobacterium bacteremia
C.   Both
D.   Neither

163. ___ Most often originate in the gastrointestinal tract
164. ___ Most often originate from upper respiratory tract
165. ___ Lower mortality rate if origin is in genitourinary tract
166. ___ Early invasion of regional veins
167. ___ Anaerobic non-sporulating gram negative bacilli
168. ___ Anaerobic gram positive bacilli
      Ref. Felner, J. N. , Dowell, V. R. : "Bacteroides" Bacteremia.
      Amer J Med, 50:787, 1971.

A.   Peripheral WBC count usually elevated
B.   Routine blood culture often positive
C.   Both
D.   Neither

169. ___ Diplococcus pneumoniae pneumonia
170. ___ Staphylococcus aureus pneumonia
171. ___ Psittacosis
172. ___ Tuberculosis
173. ___ Hemophilus influenzae pneumoniae in adults
      Ref. Carpenter, C. J. , Jr. , Mulholland, J. H. : Pneumonia in The
      Principles and Practice of Medicine, 17th Ed, Chap 73, Appleton-
      Century-Crofts, New York, 1968, pp. 723-736.

A.   Klebsiella sp.
B.   Serratia sp.
C.   Both
D.   Neither

174. ___ Sensitive to cephalothin
175. ___ Resistant to cephalothin
176. ___ Sensitive to colistin
177. ___ Resistant to colistin
      Ref. Ramirez, M. J. : Differentiation of Klebsiella - Enterobacter
      (Aerobacter) - Serratia by Biochemical Tests and Antibiotic
      Susceptibility. Appl Microbiol, 16:1548, 1971.

A.   Gram negative bacillary bacteremia
B.   Staphylococcal sepsis
C.   Both
D.   Neither

178. ___ Alcoholism
179. ___ Sarcoid
180. ___ Convulsive disorder
181. ___ Exfoliative dermatitis
182. ___ Asthma
183. ___ Hepatic cirrhosis
      Ref. Fekety, F. R. , Cluff, L. E. : Epidemiology and Host-Parasite
      Relationships in The Principles and Practice of Medicine, 17th Ed,
      Appleton-Century-Crofts, New York, 1968, pp. 645-653.

A. Neisseria meningitidis
B. Neisseria gonorrhoeae
C. Both
D. Neither

184. ___ Meningitis
185. ___ Endocervical infection
186. ___ Fermentation of glucose
187. ___ Arthritis
188. ___ Genital vesicles
Ref. Taubin, H. L. , Landsberg, L. : Gonococcal Meningitis. New Eng
J Med, 285:504, 1971. Keys, T. F. , Hecht, R. H. , Chow, A. W. :
Endocervical Neisseria Meningitidis with Meningococcemia. New Eng
J Med, 285:505, 1971.

A. Macular eruption
B. Petechial or purpuric eruption
C. Both
D. Neither

189. ___ Chancroid
190. ___ Diphtheria
191. ___ Typhus
192. ___ Measles
193. ___ Secondary syphilis
194. ___ Tularemia
195. ___ Smallpox
Ref. Fekety, F. R. , Cluff, L. E. : The Clinical and Laboratory
Manifestations of Infectious Diseases in The Principles and Practice
of Medicine. 17th Ed, Chap 66, Appleton-Century-Crofts, New York,
1968, pp. 654-671.

IN THE FOLLOWING QUESTIONS, CHOOSE:
A. If 1, 2 and 3 are correct
B. If 1 and 3 are correct
C. If 2 and 4 are correct
D. If only 4 is correct
E. If all 4 are correct

196. THE FOLLOWING NEUROLOGIC SYNDROMES HAVE BEEN ASSOCIATED
WITH VIBRIO FETUS INFECTION:
1. Subarachnoid hemorrhage
2. Meningo-encephalitis
3. Peripheral neuropathy
4. Stroke syndrome
Ref. Gunderson, C. H. , Sack, G. E. : Neurology of Vibrio Fetus Infection.
Neurology, 21:307, 1971.

197. THE GENERA PEPTOCOCCUS AND PEPTOSTREPTOCOCCUS ARE
SENSITIVE TO:
1. Penicillin
2. Erythromycin
3. Chloramphenicol
4. Gentamicin
Ref. Pien, F. D. , Thompson, R. L. , Martin, W. J. : Clinical and
Bacteriologic Studies of Anaerobic Gram-Positive Cocci. Mayo Clin Proc,
47:251, 1972.

198.   THE GENERA PEPTOCOCCUS AND PEPTOSTREPTOCOCCUS ARE
        SENSITIVE TO:
        1. Penicillin
        2. Erythromycin
        3. Cephalothin
        4. Lincomycin
        Ref. Pien, F. D., Thompson, R. L., Martin, W. J.: Clinical and
        Bacteriologic Studies of Anaerobic Gram-Positive Cocci. Mayo Clin
        Proc, 47:251, 1972.

199.   THE CLINICAL CHARACTERISTICS OF INFECTIVE ENDOCARDITIS
        DUE TO CHLAMYDIA PSITTACI INCLUDE:
        1. Negative blood cultures
        2. Rising titers of serum complement fixing antibodies to P/LGV
            antigen
        3. Prominent vegetations on the heart valves
        4. Rising titers of serum complement fixing antibodies against
            C. burneti
        Ref. Levison, D. A. Guthrie, W., Ward, C., et al: Infective
        Endocarditis as a Part of Psittacosis. Lancet, 2:844, 1971.

200.   WHICH OF THE FOLLOWING CULTURAL RESULTS ARE COMPATIBLE
        WITH GROWTH OF FLAVOBACTERIUM MENINGOSEPTICUM?:
        1. Citrate negative
        2. Nitrate negative
        3. Gram negative rod
        4. Weakly oxidase positive
        Ref. Werthamer, S., Weiner, M.: Subacute Bacterial Endocarditis
        due to Flavobacterium Meningosepticum. Amer J Clin Path, 57:410,
        1972.

201.   WHICH OF THE FOLLOWING SYNDROMES ARE COMPATIBLE WITH
        THE DIAGNOSIS OF VIBRIOSIS?:
        1. Bacterial endocarditis and thrombophlebitis
        2. Neonatal meningitis
        3. Septic abortion
        4. Monarticular septic arthritis
        Ref. Dolev, E., Altmann, G., Padeh, B.: Vibriofetus Septicemia.
        Israel J Med Sci, 7:1188, 1971.

202.   THE FOLLOWING CLINICAL FEATURES OCCUR IN ESSENTIALLY
        ALL PATIENTS WITH ROCKY MOUNTAIN SPOTTED FEVER:
        1. Malaise
        2. Fever
        3. Maculopapular rash
        4. Generalized myalgia
        Ref. Vianna, N. J., Himman, A. R.: Rocky Mountain Spotted Fever on
        Long Island. Amer J Med, 51:725, 1971.

203.   PATIENTS SUFFERING FROM SEVERE TETANUS USUALLY HAVE:
        1. Abnormally low excretion of a water load
        2. Edema
        3. Falling packed cell volume
        4. Clinical picture of low circulating blood volume
        Ref. Holloway, R.: Fluid and Electrolyte Status in Tetanus. Lancet,
        2:1278, 1970.

204. OF THE FOLLOWING, THE MAJOR DETERMINANT IN EVALUATING
      HUMAN SERUM BACTERICIDAL CAPACITY AGAINST H.
      INFLUENZAE IS:
      1. Buffer used in the procedure
      2. Derivation of serum from healthy adults
      3. Source of isolation of the bacteria
      4. Strain of H. influenzae used
      Ref. Norden, C. W. : Variable Susceptibility of Hemophilus Influenzae,
      Type B Strains, to Serum Bactericidal Activity. Proc Soc Expl Biol Med,
      139:59, 1972.

205. INITIAL TREATMENT OF INFECTION CAUSED BY BACTEROIDES
      FRAGILIS WOULD PROPERLY INCLUDE WHICH OF THE FOLLOWING
      DRUGS?:
      1. Clindamycin
      2. Penicillin G
      3. Chloramphenicol
      4. Tetracycline
      Ref. Kislak, J. W. : The Susceptibility of Bacteroides Fragilis to 24
      Antibiotics. J Infect Dis. 125:295, 1972.

206. BOTH MENINGOCOCCAL AND GONOCOCCAL MENINGITIS ARE
      ASSOCIATED WITH:
      1. Petachiae
      2. Myocarditis
      3. Endocarditis
      4. Arthritis
      Ref. Sayeed, Z. A. , Bhaduri, U. , Howell, E. , et al: Gonococcal
      Meningitis. JAMA, 219:1731, 1972.

207. THE FOLLOWING ARE CHARACTERISTICS OF GONOCOCCAL
      TONSILLAR INFECTIONS:
      1. Lack of any characteristic signs and symptoms
      2. Most consistently associated with oro-genital contact
      3. Resistant to treatment with penicillin
      4. Almost always responds to treatment with tetracycline
      Ref. Bro-Jorgensen, A. , Jensen, T. : Gonococcal Tonsillar Infection.
      Brit Med J, 4:660, 1971.

208. BACTEROIDES MELANINOGENICUS CAN BE EXPECTED TO BE
      SENSITIVE TO:
      1. Erythromycin
      2. Penicillin
      3. Chlortetracycline
      4. Chloramphenicol
      Ref. Werner, H. , Pulverer, G. , Reichertz, C. : The Biochemical
      Properties and Antibiotic Susceptibility of Bacteroides Melaninogenicus.
      Med Microbiol Immunol, 157:3, 1971.

209. ERWINIA SPECIES ARE USUALLY RESISTANT TO WHICH OF THE
      FOLLOWING ANTIBIOTICS?:
      1. Ampicillin
      2. Cephalothin
      3. Tetracycline
      4. Gentamicin
      Ref. Meyers, B. R. , Bottone, E. , Hirschman, S. , et al: Infections
      Caused by Microorganisms of the Genus Erwinia. Ann Int Med, 76:9, 1972.

210.   WHICH OF THE FOLLOWING CULTURAL REACTIONS ARE
        CHARACTERISTIC OF ERWINIA SPECIES?:
        1. Triple sugar iron - acid slant/acid butt
        2. Symplasma formation
        3. Yellow pigment production
        4. Produce ornithine decarboxylase
        Ref. Meyers, B. R. Bottone, E., Hirschman, S. Z., et al: Infections
        Caused by Microorganisms of the Genus Erwinia. Ann Int Med,
        76:9, 1972.

211.   THE FOLLOWING EVENTS ARE OF CRITICAL IMPORTANCE IN THE
        PATHOGENESIS OF EXPERIMENTAL RETROGRADE E. COLI
        PYELONEPHRITIS IN THE RAT:
        1. Bacteremia
        2. Water deprivation
        3. Abnormal pyelovenous communications
        4. Volume of inoculum refluxed to the renal pelvis
        Ref. Fierer, J., Talner, L., Braude, A. I.: Bacteremia in the
        Pathogenesis of Retrograde E. Coli Pyelonephritis in the Rat.
        Amer J Pathol, 64:443, 1971.

212.   PASTURELLA MULTOCIDA INFECTION MAY CAUSE:
        1. Infected cat bites
        2. Meningitis
        3. Brain abscess
        4. Mastoiditis
        Ref. Schwartz, M., Kunz, L.: Pasturella Multocida Infections in Man.
        N Eng J Med, 261:889, 1959.

213.   SKIN MANIFESTATIONS ASSOCIATED WITH M. PNEUMONIAE
        INFECTIONS INCLUDE:
        1. Erythema nodosum
        2. Erythema multiforme
        3. Papulovesicular eruptions
        4. Petechiae
        Ref. Teisch, J. A., Shapiro, L., Walzer, R. A.: Vesiculopustular
        Eruption with Mycoplasma Infection. JAMA, 211:1694, 1970.

214.   RICKETTSIAL DISEASE SYNDROMES WHICH OCCUR NATURALLY IN
        THE UNITED STATES ARE:
        1. Rocky Mountain spotted fever
        2. Brill's disease
        3. Murine typhus
        4. Rickettsial pox
        Ref. Hattwick, M. A.: Rocky Mountain Spotted Fever in the United States,
        1920-1970. J Infect Dis, 124:112, 1971.

215.   COMMON SOURCES OF GRAM NEGATIVE BACILLARY BACTEREMIA
        IN HOSPITALIZED PATIENTS ARE:
        1. Urinary tract infection
        2. Biliary tract disease
        3. Appendicitis
        4. Pneumonia
        Ref. Castleman, B. F.: Case Records of the Massachusetts General
        Hospital. New Eng J Med, 285:220, 1971.

216. SOME COMMONLY CITED REASONS WHY GONORRHEA CONTINUES
      TO INCREASE ARE:
      1. Very brief incubation period
      2. Asymptomatic nature of the infection in women
      3. Lack of acquired immunity
      4. Decreasing sensitivity of the gonococcus to penicillin
      Ref. Lucas, J. B.: Gonococcal Resistance to Antibiotics. South Med Bull,
      59:22, 1971.

217. A PHARYNGEAL MEMBRANE WHICH LEAVES A BLEEDING SURFACE
      WHEN PULLED AWAY MAY BE SEEN IN:
      1. Diphtheria
      2. Infectious mononucleosis
      3. Vincent's angina
      4. Oral candidiasis
      Ref. McCloskey, R. V.: Rhinopharyngitis in Science and Practice of
      Clinical Medicine, Ed by Sanford, J. P., Fudenberg, H. (in press)

218. SATISFACTORY THERAPY OF ACUTE UNCOMPLICATED PRIMARY
      URINARY TRACT INFECTIONS IN NONDIABETIC ADULT WOMEN CAN
      USUALLY BE ACCOMPLISHED USING:
      1. Sulfisoxazole
      2. Triple sulfa preparations
      3. Ampicillin
      4. Tetracycline
      Ref. Marr, J. J.: Recent Developments in the Treatment of Infectious
      Diseases. Miss Med, April, 1971, p. 241.

219. ACCEPTED INDICATIONS FOR AORTIC VALVULAR SURGERY IN A
      PATIENT WITH BACTERIAL ENDOCARDITIS AND AORTIC INSUF-
      FICIENCY INCLUDE:
      1. Severe congestive heart failure
      2. Multiple episodes of arterial embolization
      3. No effective bactericidal antibiotic for the infecting organism
      4. Cardiac arrhythmia
      Ref. Griffin, F. M., Jones, G., Cobbs, C.: Aortic Insufficiency in
      Bacterial Endocarditis. Ann Int Med, 76:23, 1972.

220. VIBRIO PARAHEMOLYTICUS CAN BE IDENTIFIED BY THE FOLLOWING
      CULTURAL CHARACTERISTICS:
      1. Fails to grow well on eosinmethylene blue agar
      2. Oxidase positive
      3. Halophilic
      4. Kliglers iron agar: alkaline slant, acid butt, no gas, no H_2S production
      Ref. Dolev, E., Altmann, G., Padeh, B.: Vibrio Fetus Septicemia.
      Israel J Med Sci, 7:1188, 1971.

221. PURIFIED M PROTEIN ISOLATED FROM GROUP A STREPTOCOCCI
      HAS BEEN SHOWN TO CAUSE WHICH OF THE FOLLOWING CYTOTOXIC
      REACTIONS?:
      1. Platelet aggregation
      2. Polymorphonuclear leukocyte vacuolation
      3. Loss of phagocytic ability by polymorphonuclear leukocytes
      4. Platelet fusion
      Ref. Beachey, E. H., Stollerman, G. H.: Toxic Effects of Streptococcal
      M Protein on Platelets and Polymorphonuclear Leukocytes in Human Blood.
      J Exp Med, 134:351, 1971.

222.   SINGLE ORGANISM INFECTION WITH B. FRAGILIS IS COMMON IN:
       1. Appendicitis
       2. Peritonitis
       3. Pleural empyema
       4. Lung abscess
       Ref. Werner, H., Pulverer, G.: Incidence and Medical Significance of
       Bacteroides and Sphaerophorus Strains. Deutsch Med Wschr, 96:1325,
       1971.

223.   WHICH OF THE FOLLOWING ANIMALS MAY SERVE AS A RESERVOIR
       FOR THE PLAGUE BACILLUS?:
       1. Squirrel
       2. Cat
       3. Rabbit
       4. Dog
       Ref. Rust, J. H., Miller, B. E., Bahmanyar, M., et al: The Role of
       Domestic Animals in the Epidemiology of Plague. J Infec Dis,
       124:527, 1971.

224.   THE FOLLOWING ARE CHARACTERISTICS OF LISTERIA MONO-
       CYTOGENES MENINGITIS:
       1. Most patients are males
       2. Organism unlikely to be seen on gram stain of cerebrospinal fluid
       3. Clinical signs and symptoms are the same as other bacterial
           central nervous system infections
       4. Organism rarely found in the blood
       Ref. Lavetter, A., et al: Meningitis due to Listeria Monocytogenes.
       New Eng J Med, 285:598, 1971.

225.   WHICH OF THE FOLLOWING ARE CHARACTERISTICS OF P.
       AERUGINOSA ISOLATED FROM DISTILLED WATER IN HOSPITALS?:
       1. P. aeruginosa actually grows in distilled water
       2. P. aeruginosa grows to greater concentrations in mist therapy
           water compared to distilled water
       3. Organisms freshly isolated from water are more resistant to
           physico-chemical stresses than subcultured organisms
       4. Organisms may persist in mist therapy water for as long as 40 days
       Ref. Favero, M. S., et al: Pseudomonas aeruginosa: Growth in Distilled
       Water from Hospitals. Science, 173:836, 1971.

226.   THE EPIDEMIC POTENTIAL OF AN INFECTIOUS DISEASE IS
       DETERMINED BY:
       1. The number of susceptibles in the population
       2. The size of the population
       3. Nature and frequency of contacts among the susceptibles
       4. Proportion of the population immune
       Ref. Fox, J. P., Elveback, L., Scott, W., et al: Herd Immunity:
       Basic Concepts and Relevance to Public Health Immunization Practices.
       Amer J Epidem, 94:179, 1971.

227.   THE MOST COMMON ETIOLOGIC AGENTS RESPONSIBLE FOR FATAL
       INFECTIONS IN CHILDREN WITH LEUKEMIA ARE:
       1. S. aureus
       2. P. aeruginosa
       3. S. fecalis
       4. C. albicans
       Ref. Hughes, W. T.: Fatal Infections in Childhood Leukemia. Am J Dis
       Child, 122:283, 1971.

228. WHICH OF THE FOLLOWING ARE CHARACTERISTICS OF RE-
CRUDESCENT MELIOIDOSIS?:
1. Latent period from original infection to recrudesence may be several
years
2. Recrudesence may follow surgery
3. Sepsis may be the clinical presentation when the disease reactivates
4. May occur in the absence of primary disease identifiable as
melioidosis
Ref. Sanford, J. P., Moore, W. L.: Recrudescent Melioidosis: A
Southeast Asian Legacy. Am Rev Resp Dis, 104:452, 1971.

229. THE FOLLOWING ARE CHARACTERISTICS OF ECYTHYMA
GANGRENOSUM:
1. Each lesion progresses through edema, erythema, hemorrhagic
bullae, frank necrosis
2. May go through above sequence in less than 12 hours
3. Vein wall is invaded by bacteria
4. Intima of subdermal veins not involved
Ref. Dorff, G. J., et al: Pseudomonas Septicemia. Arch Int Med,
128:591, 1971.

230. THE SELECTIVITY OF THAYER-MARTIN MEDIUM FOR GONOCOCCI IS
DUE TO THE FOLLOWING ANTIBIOTICS:
1. Vancomycin
2. Colistin
3. Nystatin
4. Neomycin
Ref. Ellner, P. D.: Diagnosis of Gonococcal Infection. Clin Med,
78:16, 1971.

231. THE FOLLOWING AGENTS ARE RECOMMENDED IN THE INITIAL
THERAPY OF GRAM NEGATIVE BACILLEMIA ASSOCIATED WITH
PETECHIAE, GASTROINTESTINAL BLEEDING AND THROMBO-
CYTOPENIA:
1. Antibiotics
2. Epsilon-aminocaproic acid
3. Heparin
4. Intravenous fibrinogen
Ref. Yoshikawa, T., Tanaka, K. R., Guze, L. B.: Infection and
Disseminated Intravascular Coagulation. Medicine, 50:237, 1971.

232. A BURN UNIT EXPERIENCED AN OUTBREAK OF BURN INFECTIONS
DUE TO A SPECIES OF PSEUDOMONAS AERUGINOSA. AN
EPIDEMIOLOGIC INVESTIGATION WOULD MOST LIKELY INCRIMINATE
WHICH OF THE FOLLOWING AS SOURCES OF THIS ORGANISM?:
1. Ward air
2. Hands of ward staff
3. Antibiotic containing dressing cream
4. Hydrotherapy tank
Ref. Stone, H. H., Kolb, L. D.: The Evolution and Spread of Gentamicin-
Resistant Pseudomonads. J Trauma, 11:586, 1971.

233. THE FOLLOWING STATEMENTS COMPARE INFECTIVE ENDO-
CARDITIS IN THE ANTIBIOTIC ERA TO INFECTIVE ENDOCARDITIS
IN THE PREANTIBIOTIC ERA. WHICH OF THE STATEMENTS
CORRECTLY DESCRIBES INFECTIVE ENDOCARDITIS IN THE
ANTIBIOTIC ERA?:
   1. Improved survival rates in enterococcal endocarditis
   2. Decreasing involvement of the aortic valve
   3. Younger mean age of patients
   4. Essentially unchanged percentage of patients with history of
      clinically documented rheumatic fever
   Ref. Cherubin, C. E. , Neu, H. C. : Infective Endocarditis at the
   Presbyterian Hospital in New York City from 1938-1967. Amer J Med,
   51:83, 1971.

234. WHICH OF THE FOLLOWING STATEMENTS CONCERNING ENTERO-
PATHIC E. COLI ARE CORRECT?:
   1. Can colonize the jejunum
   2. Produce a heat stable enterotoxin
   3. Most often produce diarrhea in children less than 6 months of age
   4. Stable antibiotic sensitivity pattern
   Ref. South, M. A. : Enteropathogenic Escherichia Coli Disease: New
   Developments and Perspectives. J Pediat, 79:1, 1971.

235. CLOSTRIDIUM WELCHII MENINGITIS HAS BEEN ASSOCIATED WITH
THE FOLLOWING UNDERLYING ILLNESSES:
   1. Skull fracture
   2. Penetrating head wounds
   3. Brain abscess
   4. Duodenal ulcer
   Ref. Mackay, N. N. S. , Gruneberg, R. N. , Harries, B. J. : Primary
   Clostridium Welchii Meningitis. Brit MJ, 1:591, 1971.

236. WHICH OF THE FOLLOWING STATEMENTS CONCERNING
SHIGELLOSIS IS TRUE?:
   1. Shigella stool IgA concentration is higher than in normal stool
   2. Shigella stool IgM is no higher than normal stool IgM concentration
   3. Coproantibodies in shigella stool may be IgM, IgA or IgG
   4. There is no evidence that coproantibodies play any role in recovery
      from shigellosis
   Ref. Reed, W. P. , Williams, R. C. , Jr. : Intestinal Immunoglobulins
   in Shigellosis. Gastroenterology, 61:35, 1971.

237. ERWINIA SPECIES RARELY CAUSE DISEASE IN MAN ALTHOUGH
BACTEREMIA, WOUND INFECTIONS, AND BRAIN ABSCESS HAVE BEEN
REPORTED. ERWINIA SPECIES ARE USUALLY SENSITIVE TO:
   1. Ampicillin
   2. Cephalothin
   3. Penicillin
   4. Gentamicin
   Ref. Wechsler, A. , Bottone, E. , Lasser, R. , et al: Brain Abscess
   Caused by an Erwinia Species. Amer J Med, 51:680, 1971.

EACH GROUP OF ITEMS CONSISTS OF A LIST OF LETTERED HEADINGS
FOLLOWED BY A LIST OF NUMBERED WORDS OR PHRASES. FOR
EACH NUMBERED WORD OR PHRASE, SELECT THE ONE HEADING
MOST CLOSELY RELATED TO IT:

A. Coal miners' silicosis
B. Infected pulmonary infarction
C. Infected bronchogenic cyst
D. Polyarteritis nodosa
E. Caplan's syndrome

238. ___ Occupational history, positive rheumatoid disease serologic test
239. ___ Conglomerate masses with cavitation
240. ___ Peripheral density with atelectasis
241. ___ Usually single lesion
242. ___ Often multiple cavities
Ref. Wagley, P. F. , Johns, C. J. , Cader, G. , et al: Bronchopulmonary
Suppuration, Chap 40 in The Principles and Practice of Medicine,
Appleton-Century-Crofts, New York, 1968, pp. 402-410.

A. Shigellae
B. Vibrio cholera
C. Escherichia coli
D. Clostridium perfringens
E. Salmonellae
F. Staphylococci

243. ___ Marked abdominal pain
244. ___ 4-8 hour incubation period
245. ___ Bacteremia
246 ___ Hypokalemia
247. ___ Seizures; meningismus
248. ___ Usually restricted to newborn
Ref. Grody, G. F. , Keusch, G. T. : Pathogenesis of Bacterial Diarrheas.
NEJ Med, 285:831, 1971.

BIOCHEMICAL MECHANISM OF ANTIBIOTIC RESISTANCE:

A. Beta-lactamase
B. Acetylation
C. Phosphorylation
D. Phosphorylation or adenylation
E. Change in permeability of cell wall
F. Unknown

249. ___ Chloramphenicol
250. ___ Penicillin
251. ___ Streptomycin
252. ___ Kanamycin
253. ___ Cephalosporin
254. ___ Gentamicin
255. ___ Tetracycline
256. ___ Sulfonamide
257. ___ Neomycin
Ref. Neu, H. C. : Resistance of Gram Negative Bacteria to Antimicrobial
Agents in Gram Negative Sepsis, Sanford, J. P. , (ed). Med Com,
New York, N. Y. 1972, p. 26.

A. Requires strict isolation in hospital
B. Respiratory isolation
C. Protective isolation
D. Enteric isolation
E. Requires wound and skin precautions in hospital
F. Requires discharge precautions
G. Requires blood precautions only

258. ___ Malaria
259. ___ Diphtheria
260. ___ Chicken pox
261. ___ Hepatitis
262. ___ Mucocutaneous syphilis
263. ___ Impetigo
264. ___ Pemphigus
Ref. Isolation Techniques for Hospitals, Public Health Service, Publication 2054, Brachmann, P. S., (ed), U. S. Govt Printing Office, Washington, 197

THE FOLLOWING QUESTIONS RELATE TO TYPICAL ANTIMICROBIAL SENSITIVITIES OF URINARY PATHOGENS:

A. E. coli
B. Klebsiella sp.
C. Enterococcus
D. Enterobacter

265. ___ Resistant to ampicillin, carbenicillin; sensitive to kanamycin, cephalothin
266. ___ Resistant to ampicillin, cephalothin, sensitive to carbenicillin, gentamicin
267. ___ Sensitive to most antibiotics
268. ___ Resistant to kanamycin, gentamicin, sensitive to ampiciliin
Ref. Wallace, J. F., Petersdorf, R. G.: Urinary Tract Infections. Postgrad Med, 50:138, 1971.

A. Gas gangrene
B. Necrotizing fasciitis
C. Synergistic bacterial gangrene

269. ___ Group A beta hemolytic streptococcus
270. ___ Slow onset
271. ___ Following needle punctures
272. ___ Thrombosis of small blood vessels
273. ___ Extensive muscle death
Ref. Andrews, E. C., Rockwood, C. A., Cruz, A. B.: Unusual Surgical Infections. Texas Med, 65:44, 1969.

A. Paronychia
B. Terminal pulp infection of the finger
C. Palmar infection
D. Acute cellulitis of the hand
E. Tendon sheath infection of the digit

274. ___ Lymphangitis usually absent
275. ___ Extreme pain on extension of the finger
276. ___ Puncture wound often present
277. ___ Lymphangitis usually present
278. ___ Subcuticular pus
Ref. Sneddon, J.: The Care of Hand Infections. Baltimore, Williams & Wilkins Co., 1970.

THE FOLLOWING QUESTIONS REFER TO INFECTION FOLLOWING
KIDNEY TRANSPLANTATION:

A. Gram negative bacilli
B. Urinary tract
C. Wound
D. Gram positive bacilli
E. Cytomegalovirus
F. Urinary extravasation

279. ___ Most common site of infection
280. ___ Most common etiologic organism
281. ___ Second most common site of infection
282. ___ More likely to respond to treatment
283. ___ Often causes wound infection
284. ___ Acute hemorrhagic pancreatitis
Ref. Burgos-Calderon, R., Pankey, G. A., Figueroa, J. E.: Infection
in Kidney Transplantation. Surgery, 70:334, 1971.

A. Pertussis
B. Parapertussis
C. Both pertussis and parapertussis
D. Neither pertussis and parapertussis

285. ___ Most cases occur in children 3-5 years old
286. ___ Only a few cases in children more than 10 years old
287. ___ Infections without symptoms quite common
288. ___ Ratio of clinical/subclinical infections about 75%
289. ___ Epidemic peaks every 4 years
Ref. Lautrop, H.: Epidemics of parapertussis. Lancet, 1:1195, 1971.

A. Pseudomonas aeruginosa
B. E. coli
C. Proteus sp.
D. Bacteroides sp.

290. ___ Pyelonephritis and pneumonia
291. ___ Bacillary infiltration of arterial walls
292. ___ Lobar pneumonia
293. ___ Uterine infection with large empyema
294. ___ Reversal of diurnal temperature curve
Ref. Lerner, A. M., Federman, J. M.: Gram Negative Bacillary
Pneumonia. J Infect Dis, 124:425, 1971.

A. Klebsiella sp.
B. Serratia sp.
C. Characteristic of both klebsiella sp. and serratis sp.
D. Not characteristic of either klebsiella sp. or serratia sp.

295. ___ Non-motile
296. ___ Motile
297. ___ Ornithine decarboxylase positive
298. ___ Citrate positive
299. ___ Usually resistant to colistimethate
300. ___ Urinary pathogen only
Ref. Edmondson, E. B., Sanford, J. P.: The Klebsiella-Enterobacter
(Aerobacter) Serratia Group. Medicine, 46:323, 1967.

A. Gas gangrene
B. Synergistic bacterial gangrene
C. Fournier's gangrene
D. Necrotizing fasciitis

301. ___ S. aureus and microaerophilic nonhemolytic streptococcus
302. ___ Edema with crepitation
303. ___ Usually limited to scrotum, penis and perineum
304. ___ Skin may be anesthetic
305. ___ Group A β hemolytic streptococcus
306. ___ Hypocalcemia
      Ref. Andrews, E. C., Rockwood, C. A., Cruz, A. B.: Unusual Surgical
      Infections. Texas Medicine, 65:44, 1969. Werner, J., Falk, M.: Acute
      Gangrene of the Scrotum in an 8 Year-Old. J Ped, 65:133, 1964.

A. Leukemia
B. Hodgkin's disease
C. Alcoholism
D. Narcotic addiction
E. Congenital heart disease

307. ___ Tuberculosis
308. ___ Lung abscess
309. ___ Listerial meningitis
310. ___ Brain abscess
311. ___ Tetanus
      Ref. Fekety, F. R., Cluff, L. E.: Epidemiology and Host-Parasite
      Relationships, Chap 65 in The Principles and Practice of Medicine,
      17th Ed, Appleton-Century-Crofts, New York, 1968, pp. 645-653.

A. Diplococcus pneumoniae pneumonia
B. Staphylococcus aureus pneumonia
C. Mycoplasma pneumoniae pneumonia
D. Coccidioides immitis pneumonia
E. Francisella tularensis pneumonia

312. ___ Multiple chills
313. ___ Bullous myringitis
314. ___ Usually single shaking chill at onset of disease
315. ___ Cutaneous ulcer
316. ___ Erythema nodosum
      Ref. Carpenter, C. J., Jr., Mulholland, J. H.: Pneumonia in The
      Principles and Practice of Medicine, 17th Ed, Chap 73, Appleton-
      Century-Crofts, New York, 1968, pp. 723-736

DISCS CONTAINING VARIOUS ANTIBIOTICS ARE USED IN THE LABORATORY TO OBTAIN PURE CULTURES OF CERTAIN PATHOGENS WHEN MIXED WITH OTHER ORGANISMS. THE FOLLOWING QUESTIONS RELATE TO THIS TECHNIQUE:

A. Bacitracin - 10 units/disc
B. Kanamycin - 30 μg/disc
C. Neomycin - 30 μg/disc
D. Nystatin - 100 units/disc
E. Sulfadimethoxine - 1 μg/disc
F. Penicillin - 10 units/disc

317. ___ Isolation of H influenzae on chocolate agar
318. ___ Isolate beta hemolytic from alpha hemolytic streptococci
319. ___ Isolate B.pertussis on Bordet-Gengou agar
320. ___ Separate yeasts from bacteria
321. ___ Isolate beta hemolytic streptococci from staphylococci
322. ___ Isolate bacteroides from other organisms in anaerobic cultures

Ref. Vera, H.: Quality Control in Diagnostic Microbiology. Health Lab Sci, 8:176, 1971.

FOR EACH OF THE FOLLOWING MULTIPLE CHOICE QUESTIONS,
SELECT THE ONE MOST APPROPRIATE ANSWER:

323. AN ANTIVIRAL EFFECT OF RIFAMPICIN HAS BEEN DEMONSTRATED
IN HUMAN INFECTION WITH:

A. Vaccinia virus   D. Dengue virus
B. Influenza virus   E. Coronaviruses
C. Parainfluenza virus

Ref. Moshkowitz, A., Goldblum, N., Heller, E.: Studies on the
Antiviral Effect of Rifampicin in Volunteers. Nature, 229:422, 1971.

324. THE MOST COMMON CARDIAC ABNORMALITY IN PATIENTS DYING
OF VIRAL HEPATITIS IS:

A. Subendocardial lymphocytic infiltration
B. Myocardial fatty degeneration
C. Subendocardial edema
D. Epicardial lymphocytic infiltration
E. Widespread petechial hemorrhage

Ref. Bell, H.: Cardiac Manifestations of Viral Hepatitis. JAMA,
218:387, 1971.

325. AN ANTIVIRAL ACTIVITY OF RIFAMYCIN IN VITRO HAS BEEN
DEMONSTRATED USING:

A. Influenza virus   D. Vaccinia virus
B. Parainfluenza virus   E. Dengue virus
C. Coronaviruses

Ref. Follett, E.A.C., Pennington, T.H.: Antiviral Effect of
Constituent Parts of the Rifampicin Molecule Nature, 230:117, 1971.

326. WHICH OF THE FOLLOWING ARE CONTRAINDICATIONS TO THE
ADMINISTRATION OF MEASLES VACCINE?:

A. A 6 month-old child residing in a community where there is
epidemic measles
B. A 3 year-old child with cystic fibrosis
C. A 2 year-old child under treatment for 6 months for tuberculosis
cervical lymphadenitis
D. A 14 month-old child immunized at 8 months of age with vaccine and
measles immune globulin
E. None of the above

Ref. Center for Disease Control Morbidity and Mortality, 20:387, 1971.

327. THE CAUSATIVE VIRUS CAN BE OBTAINED FROM SKIN AFFECTED
BY THE FOLLOWING EXANTHEMS:

A. Rubella   D. Herpes simplex
B. Vaccinia   E. All of the above
C. Varicella

Ref. Heggie, A.K.: Pathogenesis of the Rubella Exanthem. New Eng
J Med, 285:664, 1971.

328. ALL OF THE FOLLOWING STATEMENTS CONCERNING THE
EPIDEMIOLOGY OF RUBELLA IN THE CONTINENTAL UNITED STATES
ARE CORRECT, EXCEPT:

A. 15-20% of those over age 15 do not have antibody
B. The peak incidence is in the 5-9 year age range
C. The largest number of cases are usually reported in September
D. There is gross under-reporting of the disease
E. The usual epidemic cycle is 6-9 years

Ref. Horstmann, D.M.: Rubella: The Challenge of its Control.
J Infec Dis, 123:640, 1971.

329. THE CRITICAL ASPECT OF RABIES IMMUNE GLOBULIN (HUMAN)
(RIGH) IN POST-EXPOSURE RABIES PROPHYLAXIS IS:
A. The half time of RIGH is nearly the same as that of equine
hyperimmune serum
B. Duration of passive immunity is less with RIGH than with equine serum
C. Serum sickness is common
D. Interference with active immunity
E. Local pain on injection
Ref. Loofbourow, J. C., Cabasso, J., Roby, R. E., et al: Rabies Immune
Globulin (Human). JAMA, 217:1825, 1971.

330. WHICH OF THE FOLLOWING VIRUSES HAS RECENTLY BEEN
IMPLICATED AS A CAUSE OF HETEROPHILE ANTIBODY NEGATIVE
INFECTIOUS MONONUCLEOSIS?:
A. Cytomegalovirus
B. Epstein - Barr virus
C. Herpes virus hominis
D. Varicella-zoster virus
E. Simian virus 40
Ref. Henle, W., Henle, G., Niederman, J. C., Kemola, E., Haltia, K.:
Antibodies to Early Antigens Induced by Epstein-Barr Virus in
Infectious Mononucleosis. J Infect Dis, 124:58, 1971.

331. WHICH OF THE FOLLOWING VIRUSES HAS RECENTLY BEEN
IMPLICATED AS THE AGENT CAUSING HETEROPHILE ANTIBODY
POSITIVE INFECTIOUS MONONUCLEOSIS?:
A Cytomegalovirus
B. Epstein-Barr virus
C. Herpes virus hominis
D. Varicella- zoster virus
E. Simian virus 40
Ref. Henle, W., Henle, G., Niederman, J. C., Kemola, E., Haltia, K.:
Antibodies to Early Antigens Induced by Epstein-Barr Virus in
Infectious Mononucleosis. J Infect Dis, 124:58, 1971.

332. SUCCESSFUL HERD IMMUNITY THROUGH VACCINATION HAS BEEN
MOST EVIDENT FOR WHICH OF THE FOLLOWING VIRUSES?:
A. Measles
B. Poliomyelitis
C. Influenza
D. Rubella
E. Respiratory syncytial virus
Ref. Horstmann, D. N.: Rubella: The Challenge of its Control.
J Infec Dis, 123:640, 1971.

333. ALL OF THE STATEMENTS CONCERNING EPSTEIN-BARR VIRUS
(EBV) ARE CORRECT, EXCEPT:
A. EBV is regularly present in cultured lymphocytes from patients
with infectious mononucleosis
B. EBV persists in lymphocytes for years following infectious
mononucleosis
C. Produces infectious mononucleosis in susceptible recipients after
blood transfusion
D. Antibody to EBV appears during infectious mononucleosis
E. Antibody to EBV does not persist after infectious mononucleosis
Ref. Evans, A. S.: The Spectrum of Infections with Epstein-Barr Virus:
A Hypothesis. J Inf Dis, 124:330, 1971.

THE FOLLOWING QUESTIONS CONSIST OF PAIR OF PHRASES
DESCRIBING CONDITIONS OR QUANTITIES WHICH MAY OR MAY NOT
VARY IN RELATION TO EACH OTHER. ANSWER:
A. If increase in the first is accompanied by increase in the second or
    decrease in the first is accompanied by decrease in the second
B. If increase in the first is accompanied by decrease in the second or
    decrease in the first is accompanied by increase in the second
C. If changes in the first are independent of changes in the second

334. 1. Extent of dissemination of hematologic malignancy
      2. Severity of herpes simplex virus infection of patients with
          hematologic malignancy
      _A_   Ref. Muller, S. A., Herrmann, E. C., Winkelmann, R. K.: Herpes Simplex
      Infections in Hematologic Malignancies. Amer J Med, 52:102, 1972.

335. 1. Duration of infection with cytomegalovirus during gestation
      2. Severity of cytomegalovirus disease after birth
          Ref. Monif, G. R. G., et al: Correlation of Maternal Cytomegalovirus
      _A_ Infection During Varying Stages in Gestation with Neonatal Involvement.
      J Pediat, 80:17, 1972.

336. 1. Serum anti-neuraminidase titer
      2. Resistance to infection with influenza A_2 virus
          Ref. Slepushkin, A. N.: Neuraminidase and Resistance to Vaccination with
      _A_ Live Influenza A_2 (Hong Kong Vaccines). J Hyg, 69:571, 1971.

337. 1. Titer of serum antibody against rhinoviruses
      2. 50% human infectious dose of rhinoviruses
          Ref. Hendley, J. O., Edmondson, W. P., Gwaltney, J. M.: Relation
      _A_ Between Naturally Acquired Immunity and Infectivity of Two Rhino-
      viruses in Volunteers. J Inf Dis, 125:243, 1972.

338. 1. Serum levels of complement in viral hepatitis
      2. Titer of hepatitis-associated antigen in serum
      _B_ Ref. Alpert, E., Isselbacher, K. J., Schur, P.: The Pathogenesis of
      Arthritis Associated with Hepatitis. New Eng J Med, 285:185, 1971.

THE FOLLOWING QUESTIONS CONSIST OF A STATEMENT AND A
REASON. SELECT:
A   If both statement and reason are true and the reason is a correct
    explanation of the statement
B. If both statement and reason are true but the reason is not a correct
    explanation of the statement
C. If the statement is true but the reason is false
D. If the statement is false but the reason is true
E. If both statement and reason are false

339. _B_ Cytosine arabinoside and idoxyuridine are not very effective agents in
      the treatment of cytomegalic inclusion disease BECAUSE cyto-
      megalovirus persists following treatment with cytosine arabinoside
      and idoxyuridine
      _B_ Ref. McCracken, G. H., Luby, J. P.: Cytosine Arabinoside in the
      Treatment of Congenital Cytomegalic Inclusion Disease. J Ped,
      80:488, 1972.

340. _E_ Attempts to isolate Coxsackie or Echoviruses from the cerebrospinal
      fluid are usually nonproductive BECAUSE these viruses appear in the
      spinal fluid in less than 10% of those patients with Coxsackie virus
      or Echovirus meningitis.
      Ref. Horstmann, D.: Viral Meningitis in Textbook of Medicine. Beeson,
      P. B., McDermott, W., (Ed), W. B. Saunders Co., Philadelphia,
      1971. p. 403.

341. *A* Even when both testicles are involved by mumps virus infection, sterility seldom results BECAUSE the distribution of the inflammatory reaction is spotty.
Ref. Horstman, D.: Mumps in Textbook of Medicine. Beeson, P. B., McDermott, W., (Ed), W. B. Saunders, Philadelphia, 1971, p. 400.

342. *A* Combined measles-mumps-rubella vaccine provides an effective single vaccine immunization procedure BECAUSE a demonstrable antibody response occurs in over 90% of children receiving this vaccine.
Ref. Stokes, J. Jr., Weibel, R. E., Villarejos, V. M., et al: Trivalent Combined Measles-Mumps-Rubella Vaccine. JAMA, 218:57, 1971.

343. *A* The recombinant progeny of 2 parent influenza virus strains theoretically should not be more virulent for man than either parent strain BECAUSE progeny strains of influenza virus can only possess what has been given to them by the parent strains.
Ref. Beare, A. S., Hall, T. S.: Recombinant Influenza - A Viruses as Live Vaccines for Man. Lancet, 2:1271, 1971.

344. *C* It still is not certain whether vaccination can achieve long term protection against rubella BECAUSE antibody formation following natural disease is lower than that following vaccination.
Ref. Eichhorn, M. M., Rubella,: Will Vaccination Prevent Birth Defects. Science, 173:710, 1971.

345. *A* Rubella immunization is contra-indicated during pregnancy BECAUSE attenuated vaccine virus can infect the placenta.
Ref. Horstmann, D. M.: Rubella: The Challenge of its Control. J Infec Dis, 123:640, 1971.

346. *A* Hodgkin's disease or leukemia are absolute contraindications to vaccination BECAUSE the principle danger is the development of vaccinia gangrenosum.
Ref. Kempe, C. H.: Vaccinia in Textbook of Medicine, Ed by Beeson, P. B., McDermott, W., W. B. Saunders Co., Philadelphia, 1971, p. 392.

347. *E* Cold weather causes common colds BECAUSE exposure of volunteers to cold activates latent respiratory infections.
Ref. Jackson, G. G.: The Common Cold in Textbook of Medicine, Ed Beeson, P B., McDermott, W., W. B. Saunders, Co., Philadelphia, 1971. p. 359.

348. *A* Flucytosine should be used for the treatment of fungal infections only when the patient cannot tolerate amphotericin B BECAUSE as many as 50% of candida isolates are initially resistant to flucytosine and resistant cryptococci emerge during treatment of cryptococcal meningitis with flucytosine.
Ref. The Medical Letter, 14:29, 1972.

ANSWER THE FOLLOWING QUESTIONS ACCORDING TO THE KEY
BELOW:
A. If choice A is greater than choice B
B. If choice B is greater than choice A
C. If A and B are equal or nearly equal

349.   THE PERCENTAGE OF ADENOVIRUS INFECTIONS IN INFANTS AND
       CHILDREN WHICH RESULT IN:
       A. Minor respiratory disease
  A   B. Serious respiratory disease
       Ref. Brandt, C. D., Kim, H. W., Jeffries, B. C., et al: Infections in
       18,000 Infants and Children in a Controlled Study of Respiratory Tract
       Disease. II. Variation in Adenovirus Infections by Year and Season.
       Amer J Epidemiol, 95:218, 1972.

350.   AMOUNT OF INTERFERON PRODUCED IN RESPONSE TO INFECTION
       WITH CHIKUNGUNYA VIRUS BY PERITONEAL EXUDATE CELLS FROM:
       A. Normal mice
  A   B. Mice infected with M. lepraemurium
       Ref. Glasgow, L. A., Bullock, W. E.: Impairment of Interferon
       Production in Mice Infected with Mycobacterium Lepraemurium.
       Proc Soc Expl Biol Med, 139:492, 1972.

351.   ATTACK RATES OF SMALLPOX IN VACCINATED CONTACTS OF
       SMALLPOX WHEN:
       A. Contacts were treated with methisazone
       B. Contacts receive a placebo
  C   Ref. Heiner, G. G., Fatima, N., Russell, P. K.: Field Trials of
       Methisazone as a Prophylactic Agent Against Smallpox. Amer J Epidemiol,
       94:435, 1971.

352.   THE MIC OF IDOXURIDINE IN VITRO OF:
       A. Herpesvirus hominis, Type 1
       B. Herpesvirus hominis, Type 2
       Ref. Lerner, A. M., Bailey, E. J.: Concentrations of Idoxuridine in
       Serum, Urine and Cerebrospinal Fluid of Patients with Suspected
  B   Diagnoses of Herpesvirus Hominis Encephalitis. J Clin Invest, 51:45,
       1972.

353.   A NUMBER OF PERSONS (METROPOLITAN POPULATION) WHO WILL
       DEVELOP A CLINICAL ILLNESS WHEN INFECTED BY:
       A. Adenovirus
       B. M. pneumoniae
       Ref. Hall, C. E., Brandt, D. C., Frothingham, T. E.: The Virus
  A   Watch Program: A Continuing Surveillance of Viral Infections in
       Metropolitan New York Families. Amer J Epidemiol, 94:367, 1971.

354.   PERCENTAGE OF CHILDREN WHO PRODUCE ANTIBODIES AGAINST:
       A. Rubella virus after immunization with live measles-rubella virus
           vaccine
       B. Measles virus after immunization with live measles-rubella virus
           vaccine
  C   Ref. Villarejos, V. M., Arguedas, G. J. A., Bruynak, E. B.: Combined
       Live Measles-Rubella Virus Vaccine. J Ped, 79:599, 1971.

355. INCIDENCE OF VARICELLA-ZOSTER INFECTION OF PATIENTS WITH:
      A. Leukemia
      B. Hodgkin's disease
      Ref. Schimpff, S., Serpick, A., Stoler, B., et al: Varicella-zoster
      Infection in Patients with Cancer. Ann Intern Med, 76:241, 1972.

356. IMMUNITY TO RUBELLA AFTER:
      A. Parenteral immunization using HPV-77 rubella vaccine
      B. Intranasal immunization using RA-27/3 rubella vaccine
      Ref. Ogra, P. L, Kerr-Grant   Umana, G., et al: Antibody
      Response in Serum and Nasopharynx after Naturally Acquired and
      Vaccine-Induced Infection with Rubella Virus. New Eng J Med,
      285:1334, 1971.

357. DURATION OF FEVER IN NATURALLY OCCURRING INFLUENZA A_2
      INFECTION TREATED WITH:
      A. Placebo
      B. 1-adamantine hydrochloride 100 mgm q 12 hours
      Ref. Galbraith, A. W., Oxford, J. S., Schild, G. L., et al: Therapeutic
      Effect of 1-Adamantine Hydrochloride in Naturally Occurring Influenza
      A_2/Hong Kong Infection. Lancet, 2:113, 1971.

358. PERCENTAGE OF CHILDREN WITH RESPIRATORY SYNCITIAL VIRUS
      INFECTION WHO DEVELOP:
      A. Rales and ronchi
  C   B. Otitis
      Ref. Smith, T. F., Person, D. A., Herrmann, E. C.: Experiences in
      Laboratory Diagnosis of Respiratory Syncitial Virus Infections in
      Routine Medical Practice. Mayo Clin Proc, 46:609-612, 1971.

359. INCIDENCE OF:
      A. Parotitis in laboratory confirmed cases of mumps virus infection
      B. Cervical lymphadenitis in laboratory confirmed cases of mumps
          virus infection
  A   Ref. Person, D. A., Smith, T. F., Herrmann, E. C.: Experiences in
      Laboratory Diagnosis of Mumps Virus Infections in Routine Medical
      Practice. Mayo Clin Proc, 46:544, 1971.

360. CASE TO CASE SPREAD OF:
      A. Mycoplasma pneumonia
      B. Adenovirus pneumonia
  B   Ref. Evatt, B. L., Dowdle, W. R., Johnson, McC., et al: Epidemic
      Mycoplasma Pneumonia. New Eng J Med, 285:374, 1971.

361. THE RATE OF LOSS OF RUBELLA HI ANTIBODY IN THE SERA OF:
      A. Children with congenital rubella
      B. Mothers of children with congenital rubella
      Ref. Cooper, L. Z., Florman, A. L., Ziring, P. R., Krugman, S.:
  A   Loss of Rubella Hemagglutination Inhibition; Antibody in Congenital
      Rubella. Amer J Dis Child, 122:397, 1971.

362. PERCENTAGE OF:
      A. Normal women who have serum neutralizing antibody against Herpes
          simplex virus Type 2
  B   B. Women with cervical carcinoma who have serum neutralizing
          antibody against Herpes simplex virus Type 2
      Ref. Plummer, G., Masterson, J. G.: Herpes Simplex Virus and Cancer
      of the Cervix. Am J Obst Gyn, 111:81, 1971.

363. SERUM ANTIBODY TITERS TO MEASLES VIRUS IN:
      A. Siblings of patients with subacute sclerosing panencephalitis
      B. Siblings of controls
      Ref. Detels, R., Severs, J. L.: Measles Antibody Titers in Sibships of
C   Patients with Subacute Sclerosing Panencephalitis and Control. Lancet,
      1:177, 1972.

364. ABORTION RATE OF PREGNANT WOMEN WITH:
      A. Primary genital herpes
      B. Recurrent genital herpes
      Ref. Nahmias, A. J., Josey, W. E., Naib, Z. M., et al: Perinatal Risk
A   Associated with Maternal Genital Herpes Simplex Virus Infection.
      Am J Obst Gyn, 110:825, 1971.

365. SIDE REACTIONS FOLLOWING RUBELLA VACCINATION USING:
      A. RA 27/3 vaccine
      B. HPV-77 vaccine
B   Ref. Buser, F., Nicholas, A.: Vaccination with RA 27/3 Rubella
      Vaccine. Amer J Dis Child, 122:53, 1971.

366. INCUBATION PERIOD OF:
      A. MS1 virus hepatitis
      B. MS2 virus hepatitis
B   Ref. Krugman, S., Giles, J. P.: Viral Hepatitis: New Light on an Old
      Disease. JAMA, 212:1019, 1970.

EACH SET OF LETTERED HEADINGS IS FOLLOWED BY A NUMBERED
LIST OF WORDS OR PHRASES. ANSWER:
A. If the word or phrase is associated with A only
B. If the word or phrase is associated with B only
C. If the word or phrase is associated with A and B
D. If the word or phrase is associated with neither A nor B

      A. Mumps virus
      B. Parainfluenza virus
      C. Both
      D. Neither

367. C   Paramyxovirus
368. C   Parotitis
369. C   Bronchiolitis and croup
370. A   Recovered with greater frequency from children with respiratory
          disease compared with normal children
371. D   DNA viruses
          Ref. Foy, H. M., Cooney, M. K., Hall, C. E., et al: Isolation of Mumps
          Virus from Children with Acute Lower Respiratory Tract Disease.
          Amer J Epidemiology, 94:467, 1971.

      A. Primary influenza virus pneumonia
      B. Secondary bacterial pneumonia following influenza
      C. Both
      D. Neither

372. C   Typical onset of influenza
373. A   History of rheumatic heart disease
374. B   Afebrile period of recovery
375. A   Diffuse pulmonary abnormalities (exam and X-rays)
376. B   Elderly patient with chronic cardiopulmonary disease
          Ref. Schulman, J. L.: Influenza. Postgrad Med, 50:171, 1971.

A. Primary influenza virus pneumonia
B. Secondary bacterial pneumonia following influenza
C. Both
D. Neither

377. __A__ High mortality rate
378. __B__ Low mortality rate
379. __D__ Prominent gastrointestinal symptoms
380. __A__ Cyanosis and extreme tachypnea
381. __D__ Localized consolidation
382. __A__ Afebrile period of recovery
Ref. Schulman, J. L.: Influenza. Postgrad Med, 50:171, 1971.

A. Mumps virus infection
B. Coxsackie B virus infection
C. Both
D. Neither

383. __C__ Parotitis
384. __C__ Aseptic meningitis
385. __D__ Cause of sterility in female
386. __A__ Cause of sterility in male
387. __C__ Myocarditis
Ref. Horstmann, D.: Mumps in Textbook of Medicine, Beeson, P. B.,
McDermott, W., (Ed), W. B. Saunders Co., Philadelphia, 1971, p. 400.

A. Military recruit ARD caused by adenoviruses
B. Military recruit ARD caused by mycoplasma
C. Both
D. Neither

388. __A__ Most prominent in winter months
389. __B__ Prevalent throughout the year
390. __C__ Two to three days of fever when pneumonia appears
391. __C__ Usually lower lobe pneumonia
392. __C__ Pleural reaction and/or effusion
393. __D__ Epidemics controlled by vaccine
Ref. Wenzel, R. P., McCormick, D. P., Smith, E. P., et al: Acute
Respiratory Disease: Clinical and Epidemiologic Observations of
Military Trainees. Mil Med, 136:873, 1971.

A. Measles
B. Rubella
C. Both
D. Neither

394. __C__ Conjunctivitis
395. __B__ Sore throat
396. __D__ Leukocytosis
397. __C__ Enanthem
398. __A__ Appendicitis
399. __B__ Cataracts
Ref. Kilbourne, E. D.: Measles, Rubella in Textbook of Medicine,
Ed, Beeson, P. B., McDermott, W., W. B. Saunders Co., Philadelphia,
1971, p. 381 and p. 386.

A.　Adenovirus infections in newborn infants
B.　Adenovirus infections in young children
C.　Both
D.　Neither

400.　*B*　Mesenteric adenitis
401.　*A*　Giant cell pneumonia
402.　*C*　Coryza
403.　*D*　Croup
　　　　Ref. Jackson, G. G.: Adenoviral Infections of the Respiratory Tract
　　　　in Textbook of Medicine, Ed, Beeson, P. B., McDermott, W., W. B.
　　　　Saunders Co., Philadelphia, 1971, p. 304.

A.　Herpes simplex virus infection
B.　Vaccinia virus infection
C.　Both
D.　Neither

404.　*A*　0.1% idoxuridine instillation
405.　*D*　40% topical idoxuridine
406.　*B*　Methisazone
407.　*C*　Interferon
408.　*B*　Rifampin
　　　　Ref. The Medical Letter, 13:77-78, 1971.

A　Aseptic meningitis
B.　Encephalitis
C.　Both
D.　Neither

409.　*C*　Fever
410.　*D*　Seizures
411.　*B*　Altered state of consciousness
412.　*B*　Brain biopsy
413.　*C*　Signs of meningeal irritation
414.　*C*　Headache
　　　　Ref. Kriel, R. L.: Diagnosis and Management of Viral Encephalitis.
　　　　Postgrad Med, 50:99, 1971.

A.　Pneumonia in non-epidemic influenza years
B.　Pneumonia in epidemic influenza years
C.　Both
D.　Neither

415.　*B*　Staphylococcus aureus
416.　*C*　Association with serious underlying disease
417.　*B*　Patients generally younger
418.　*D*　Selectively affects otherwise healthy patients
419.　*C*　Pneumococcal pneumonia most frequently seen
　　　　Ref. Schwarzmann, S. W., Adler, J. L., Sullivan, R. J.: Bacterial
　　　　Pneumonia During the Hong Kong Influenza Epidemic of 1968-1969:
　　　　Experience in a City-County Hospital. Arch Int Med, 127:1037, 1971.

A. Coxsackie A viruses
B. Coxsackie B viruses
C. Both
D. Neither

420. *B* Grow readily in monkey kidney tissue cultures
421. *A* Widespread degeneration of skeletal muscle of suckling mouse
422. *B* Myocarditis in suckling mouse
423. *C* Aseptic meningitis in humans
424. *B* Orchitis in humans
425. *C* Commonly cause subclinical infections
426. *A* Herpangina
427. *D* Effective vaccines available
Ref. Zapikian, A. Z.: Coxsackie and Enteroviruses in Textbook of
Medicine, Beeson, P. B., McDermott, W., (Ed), W. B. Saunders Co.,
Philadelphia, 1971, p. 422.

IN THE FOLLOWING QUESTIONS, CHOOSE:
A   If 1, 2 and 3 are correct
B. If 1 and 3 are correct
C. If 2 and 4 are correct
D. If only 4 is correct
E. If all four are correct

428. BK VIRUS, A NEW HUMAN PAPOVAVIRUS IS:
      1. A member of the polyoma subgroup
A   2. Unrelated to SV 40
      3. Produces a hemagglutinin for human O erythrocytes
      4. Grows quickly in cell culture
Ref. Gardner, S. D., Field, A. M., Coleman, D. V., et al: New Human
Papovavirus (B. K.) Isolated from Urine After Renal Transplantation.
Lancet, 1:1253, 1971.

429. THE FOLLOWING DRUGS HAVE BEEN SHOWN TO REDUCE SYMPTOMS
      OR PREVENT INFECTION CAUSED BY INFLUENZA VIRUS A_2/HONG
      KONG:
      1. Amantadine
E   2. Rimantadine
      3. Cycloocytlamine
      4. Famotine
Ref. Togo, Y., Schwartz, A. R., Tominaga, S., et al: Cycloocytlamine
in the Prevention of Experimental Human Influenza. JAMA, 220:837,
1972.

430. THE INTRANASAL INSTILLATION OF POLY I : POLY C PRIOR TO
      VIRUS CHALLENGE OF HUMAN VOLUNTEERS WITH TYPE A_2
      INFLUENZA VIRUS RESULTS IN:
      1. High levels of nasal interferon
      2. No detectable toxic effects
C   3. Marked reduction of frequency of illness
      4. No reduction of type A_2 influenza virus shedding
Ref. Hill, D. A., Baron, S., Perkins, J. C., et al: Evaluation of an
Interferon Inducer in Viral Respiratory Disease. JAMA, 219:1179, 1972.

431. NEARLY ALL CHILDREN WITH ADENOVIRUS PNEUMONIA WILL HAVE
      THE FOLLOWING SIGNS OR SYMPTOMS:
      1. Diarrhea
      2. Cough
  C   3. Rash
      4. Fever
      Ref. Simila, S., Ylikorkala, O., Wasz-Hockert, O.: Type 7 Adenovirus
      Pneumonia. J Pediat, 79:605, 1971.

432. WHICH OF THE FOLLOWING DRUGS HAS BEEN USED WITH BENEFICIAL
      RESULTS IN THE TREATMENT OF VARICELLA-ZOSTER VIRUS
      INFECTIONS?:
      1. Emetine
      2. Idoxuridine
  C   3. Dimethylsulfoxide
      4. Cytosine arabinoside
      Ref. Hryniuk, W., Foerster, J., Shojania, M., Chow, A.: Cytarabine
      for Herpesvirus Infections. JAMA, 219:715, 1972.

433. REPORTED EXTRA-PULMONARY MANIFESTATIONS OF TYPE 7
      ADENOVIRUS PNEUMONIA INCLUDE:
      1. Encephalitis
      2. Heart failure
  E   3. Hemorrhagic phenomena
      4. Meningismus
      Ref. Simila, S.: Type 7 Adenovirus Pneumonia. J Pediatrics, 79:605,
      1971.

434. AFTER A DECLINE IN 1967-1969, THE NUMBER OF REPORTED
      MEASLES CASES INCREASED IN 1971. WHICH OF THE FOLLOWING
      WERE CHARACTERISTICS OF THESE CASE OF MEASLES?:
      1. Majority occurred in children older than 15
      2. Blacks more often affected than whites
  C   3. Number of cases highest in July and August
      4. Over 90% of previously immunized patients protected from measles
      Ref. Landrigan, P.J., Conrad, J.L.: Current Status of Measles in
      the United States. J Inf Dis, 124:620, 1972.

435. PAPOVA VIRUSES ARE SO NAMED BECAUSE THE GROUP INCLUDES:
      1. Papilloma viruses
      2. Polyoma viruses
  A   3. Simian vacuolating viruses
      4. Vaccinia virus
      Ref. Allen, D.W., Cole, P.: Viruses and Human Cancer. New Eng
      J Med, 286:70, 1971.

436. POLIOVIRUS IMMUNIZATION OF CHILDREN WITH ACUTE
      LYMPHOCYTIC LEUKEMIA IS CHARACTERIZED BY:
      1. Low IgG antibody response
      2. Normal IgA antibody response
  B   3. Absent IgM antibody response
      4. Normal antibody response
      Ref. Ogra, P.L., Sinks, L.F., Karzon, D.T.: Poliovirus Antibody
      Response in Patients with Acute Leukemia. J Pediatr, 79:444, 1971.

437. HYDATID DISEASE OF MAN OCCURS IN THE:
   1. Lung
   2. Brain
   3. Liver
E 4. Omentum
   Ref. Wolcott, M. W. , Harris, S. H. , Briggs, J. N. , et al: Hydatid
   Disease of the Lung. J Thor Cardiovasc Surg, 62:465, 1971.

438. THE FOLLOWING DISEASES ARE CAUSED BY MEMBERS OF THE
   HERPES VIRUS FAMILY:
   1. Chicken pox
   2. Fever blisters
E 3. Shingles
   4. Cytomegalic inclusion disease
   Ref. Weller, T. H. : The Cytomegaloviruses: Ubiquitous Agents with
   Protean Clinical Manifestations. New Eng J Med, 285:203, 1971.

439. DENTAL MANIFESTATIONS OF THE RUBELLA SYNDROME INCLUDE:
   1. Hyperplasia of the enamel
   2. Adentia
   3. Discoloration of enamel
D 4. Enamel hypoplasia
   Ref. Guggenheimer, J. , Nowak, A. J. , Michaels, R. H. : Dental
   Manifestations of the Rubella Syndrome. Oral Surg Med Pathol,
   32:30, 1971.

440. PRIMARY IMMUNIZATION WITH INACTIVATED POLIO VACCINE OF
   CHILDREN WITH LEUKEMIA (WHO ARE KNOWN TO BE SERONEGATIVE
   FOR POLIOVIRUS ANTIBODY PRIOR TO IMMUNIZATION) IS
   CHARACTERIZED BY:
   1. Normal production of IgG poliovirus antibody
C 2. Absent IgM poliovirus antibody production
   3. Reduced IgM poliovirus antibody production
   4. Marked reduction in IgA poliovirus antibody production
   Ref. Ogra, P. L. , Sinks, L. F. , Karzon, D. T. : Poliovirus Antibody
   Response in Patients with Acute Leukemia. J Pediatrics, 79:444, 1971.

441. CYTOMEGALOVIRUS LESIONS IN CANCER PATIENTS AT AUTOPSY ARE
   MOST OFTEN FOUND IN:
   1. Lungs
   2. Muscle
B 3. Adrenal glands
   4. Brain
   Ref. Rosen, P. , Hajdu, S. : Cytomegalovirus Inclusion Disease at
   Autopsy of Patients with Cancer. Amer J Clin Pathol, 55:749, 1971.

442. WHICH DISEASES LISTED BELOW ARE NATURALLY-OCCURRING
   DISEASES OF MAN KNOWN TO BE ASSOCIATED WITH HUMAN
   PAPOVAVIRUSES?:
   1. Papilloma
   2. Pneumonitis
B 3. Multifocal leukoencephalopathy
   4. Myocarditis
   Ref. Padgett, B. Walker, D. L. , Zurhein, G. , et al: Cultivation of
   Papova-Like Virus From Human Brain with Progressive Multifocal
   Leukoencephalopathy. Lancet 1:1257, 1971.

443. THE FOLLOWING STATEMENTS ARE TRUE IN REFERENCE TO
      PROGRESSIVE MULTIFOCAL ENCEPHALOPATHY (PML):
      1. A virus resembling SV-40 virus has been isolated from the brain
         of patients with PML
      2. The only known exposure of human beings to SV-40 virus occurred
         as a result of the use of poliovirus or adenovirus vaccines
  E   3. Most patients with PML have carcinoma or some immunologic
         abnormality
      4. SV-40 virus produces brain tumor in hamsters
      Ref. Weiner, L. P., Herndon R. M., Naragan, O., et al: Virus related
      to SV-40 in Patients with Progressive Multifocal Leukoencephalopathy
      New Eng J Med, 286:385, 1972. Black, P. H., Hirsch, M. S.: Viruses
      and Progressive Multifocal Leukoencephalopathy. New Eng J Med,
      286:429, 1972.

      EACH GROUP OF ITEMS CONSISTS OF A LIST OF LETTERED HEADINGS
      FOLLOWED BY A LIST OF NUMBERED WORDS OR PHRASES. FOR
      EACH NUMBERED WORD OR PHRASE, SELECT THE ONE HEADING
      MOST CLOSELY RELATED TO IT:

      A. Cytomegalovirus
      B. Herpes simplex virus
      C. Varicella zoster virus
      D. Toxoplasma
      E. Candida albicans

444. A   Cytosine arabinoside
445. B   Idoxuridine
446. C   Specific immune globulin
447. D   Pyrimethamine-sulfadiazine
448. E   5-fluorocytosine
      Ref. Remington, J. S.: The Compromised Host. Hospital Practice,
      7:59, 1972.

      A. Inhibition of viral entry into cell
      B. Inhibits replication of viral nucleic acid genome
      C. Inhibition of viral protein synthesis

449. B   I. U. D. R.
450. A   Amantadine
451. B   Cytosine arabinoside
452. C   Methisazone
453. C   Rifampicin
454. C   Interferon stimulators
      Ref. Hirschman, S. Z.: Approaches to Antiviral Chemotherapy.
      Amer J Med, 51:699, 1971.

      THE FOLLOWING QUESTIONS RELATE TO MECHANISMS OF AGE-
      DEPENDENT CHANGES IN SUSCEPTIBILITY TO VIRUS INFECTION OF
      THE BRAIN

      A. Coxsackie B virus
      B. Parvoviruses
      C. Sindbis virus

455. B   Postmitotic cells resistant to infection
456. A   Decrease in receptor sites in older animals
457. C   Mechanism not known
      Ref. Johnson, R. T., McFarland, H. F., Levy, S.: Age-Dependent
      Resistance to Viral Encephalitis: Studies on Infections due to Sindbis
      Virus in Mice. J Infect Dis, 125:257, 1972.

THE FOLLOWING QUESTIONS RELATE TO THE TYPE OF CYTOPATHIC EFFECT CAUSED BY A GIVEN VIRUS GROWING IN THE INDICATED CELL CULTURE:

A. Adenovirus in HeLa cells
B. Cytomegalovirus in WI-38 cells
C. Measles virus in HeLa cells
D. Influenza in monkey kidney (MK) cells

458. _B_ Localized ballooning focal lesions
459. _A_ Grape-like rounding, enlargement
460. _D_ Hemadsorption
461. _C_ Giant cell formation
    Ref. Walker, W. E., Martins, R. R., Karrels, P. A., et al: Rapid Clinical Diagnosis of Common Viruses by Specific Cytopathic Changes in Unstained Tissue Culture Roller Tubes. Amer J Clin Path, 56:384, 1971.

A. Measles virus
B. Papovavirus
C. Echovirus

462. _C_ Guillain-Barré syndrome
463. _A_ Subacute sclerosing panencephalitis
464. _B_ Progressive multifocal leukoencephalopathy
    Ref. Horta-Barbosa, L., Fuccillo, D. A., Sever, J. L.: Chronic Viral Infections of the Central Nervous System. JAMA, 218:1185, 1971.

A. Normal cerebrospinal fluid
B. Enterovirus meningitis
C. Mumps meningitis
D. Bacterial meningitis

	TOTAL PROTEIN	IgG	Mg/100ml IgA	IgM
465. _B_	30-105	1-8	.2-1.0	0
466. _A_	15-60	.8-3.5	0	0
467. _D_	85-920	4-120	.5-40	.5-16
468. _C_	25-130	2-17	.15-2.4	.9-3.8

Ref. Kaldor, J., Ferris, A. A.: Immunoglobulin Levels in Cerebrospinal Fluid in Viral and Bacterial Meningitis. Med J Austral, 2:1206, 1969.

A. C particles
B. B particles
C. Hodgkin's disease
D. Human viruses which can cause cancer in other mammals
E. Common wart

469. _B_ Virus particles of mammary tumors
470. _A_ Virus particles of animal leukemias
471. _D_ Adenoviruses
472. _C_ Herpesvirus hominis
473. _E_ Papovaviruses
    Ref. Allen, D. W., Cole, P.: Viruses and Human Cancer. New Eng J Med, 286:70, 1972.

A. Soluble (S) antigen of influenza virus
B. Type specific (V) antigen of influenza virus
C. Infectivity of influenza virus
D. Filamentous form of influenza virus

474. *D* Deficient in ribonucleoprotein
475. *A* Virus ribonucleoprotein
476. *C* Neuraminidase activity
477. *B* Hemagglutinin or neuraminidase
Ref. Rose, H. M.: Influenza: The Agent. Hospital Practice, August, 1971, p. 49.

A. General biological property of interferons
B. Prevents action of interferon
C. Production of interferon
D. Infection characteristically produces large amounts of interferon
E. Infection characteristically produces small amounts of interferon

478. *C* Statalon
479. *A* Not antigenic
480. *D* Arboviruses
481. *E* Adenoviruses
482. *B* Actinomycin D
Ref. Finter, N. B., Bucknell, R. A.: Interferon in Recent Advances in Pharmacology, Chap 16, Ed, Robson, J. M., Stacey, R. S., Little Brown & Co., Boston, 1968, pp. 429-448

A. Methisazone
B. 5 - iodo - 2 - deoxyuridine
C. Amantadine hydrochloride
D. Puromycin

483. *B* Herpes simplex keratitis
484. *A* Smallpox
485. *D* Inhibition of coat protein synthesis
486. *C* Influenza
487. *A* Inhibits late stage of viral assembly
488. *C* Blocks virus penetration
Ref. Sadler, P. W.: Chemotherapy of Virus Diseases in Recent Advances in Pharmacology, 4th Ed., Robson, J. M., Stacey, R. S., Little, Brown & Co., Boston, 1968, Chap 15, pp. 411-428.

A. Coryza
B. Pharyngitis
C. Croup
D. Bronchitis
E. Pneumonia

489. *D* Coxsackie A6 virus
490. *A* Coxsackie A 21 virus
491. *E* Influenza A, B virus
492. *C* Parainfluenza virus
493. *D* Respiratory syncitial virus
Ref. Jackson, G. G.: Nonbacterial Pharyngitis, Laryngitis, and Bronchitis in Textbook of Medicine, Ed, Beeson, P. B., McDermott, W., W. B. Saunders Co., Philadelphia, 1971, p. 362.

A. Lasting immunity with epidemic disease among susceptibles
B. Transient specific immunity
C. Inadequate antibody response from natural infection (children)
D. Mutagenic variation in the prevalent strains of virus
E. Multiple distinct types of virus simultaneously present
F. Production of latent infection

494. E B Rhinoviruses
495. F Herpesvirus hominis
496. C Respiratory syncytial virus
497. D Influenza A, B virus
498. A Measles virus

Ref. Jackson, G. G.: Nonbacterial Pharyngitis, Laryngitis, and Bronchitis in <u>Textbook of Medicine</u>, Ed., Beeson, P. B., McDermott, W., W. B. Saunders, Philadelphia, 1971, p. 362.

FOR EACH OF THE FOLLOWING MULTIPLE CHOICE QUESTIONS, SELECT THE ONE MOST APPROPRIATE ANSWER:

499. WHICH OF THE FOLLOWING ALLOWS THE PHYSICIAN TO EXCLUDE ACTIVE PULMONARY TUBERCULOSIS?:
    A. Positive Mantoux test, negative sputum smear, negative sputum culture
    B. Negative Mantoux test, negative sputum smear, negative sputum culture
    C. Positive Mantoux test, positive sputum smear, negative sputum culture
    D. Negative Mantoux test, positive sputum smear, negative sputum culture
    E. None of the above
    Ref. Elliott, H. E., Forkner, C. E., Houk, V. N., et al: Tuberculosis. Patient Care, p. 155, October, 1971.

500. SARCOID GRANULOMAS ARE MORPHOLOGICALLY AND HISTO-CHEMICALLY IDENTICAL WITH THOSE PRODUCED BY OR FOUND IN:
    A. Kveim test
    B. Farmer's lung
    C. Chronic beryllium disease
    D. Crohn's disease
    E. All of the above
    Ref. Jones-Williams, W.: Pathology of Sarcoid. Hospital Medicine, 2:21, 1967.

501. THE MOST COMMON PHYSICAL FINDING IN TUBERCULOUS PERITONITIS IS:
    A. Enlarged lymph nodes
    B. Abdominal mass
    C. Hepatomegaly
    D. Ascites
    E. Fever
    Ref. Borhanmanesh, F., Hekmat, K., Vaezzadeh, K., et al: Tuberculosis Peritonitis. Ann Intern Med, 76:567, 1972.

502. WHICH OF THE FOLLOWING IS CONSIDERED A JUSTIFIABLE INDICATION FOR SURGERY IN CHILDHOOD PULMONARY TUBERCU-LOSIS?:
    A. Thin-walled residual cavity - sputum negative
    B. Fibronodular residual - sputum negative
    C. Residual disease - sputum positive after 18 months of treatment
    D. Bronchial obstruction - sputum negative
    E. Residual pleural tuberculosis
    Ref. Feltis, J. M., Campbell, D.: Changing Role of Surgery in the Treatment of Pulmonary Tuberculosis in Children. Chest, 61:101, 1972.

503. A SMALL NUMBER OF PATIENTS CONTINUE TO DIE FROM TUBERCULOSIS IN A SHORT PERIOD OF TIME - ONE YEAR OR LESS. THESE DEATHS CAN BE MAINLY ATTRIBUTED TO:
    A. Massive pulmonary hemorrhage
    B. Delay by the physician in making the diagnosis
    C. Progressive disease due to antibiotic-resistant M. tuberculosis
    D. Delay by the patient in seeking care
    E. Post surgical deaths
    Ref. Aho, K., Jansson, S., Patiala, J.: Tuberculosis Deaths in Subjects Under Age 50 with Short Disease Histories. Scand J Resp Dis, 52:19, 1971.

504. ASSUME THAT A TUBERCULOUS PATIENT WITH MODERATELY
      ADVANCED DISEASE IS TREATED FOR 10 WEEKS WITH THE FOL-
      LOWING DRUG REGIMENS IN RECOMMENDED DOSES. ALL ORGAN-
      ISMS ARE SENSITIVE TO THE DRUGS LISTED. WHICH OF THESE
      REGIMENS WOULD BE EXPECTED TO CONVERT THE SPUTUM TO
      NEGATIVE (i. e. , NO MYCOBACTERIA PRESENT BY SMEAR OR
      CULTURE) IN 75% OF THE CASES?:
      A. Streptomycin - isoniazid - ethambutol
      B. Rifampin - isoniazid - ethambutol
      C. Rifampin - isoniazid
      D. All of the above
      Ref. Newman, R. , Doster, B. , Murray, F. J. , et al: Rifampin in
      Initial Treatment of Pulmonary Tuberculosis. Am Rev Resp Dis,
      103:461, 1971.

505. WHICH OF THE FOLLOWING ESTABLISH THE DIAGNOSIS OF
      PULMONARY CANDIDOSIS?:
      A. Detection of C. albicans by culture of sputum
      B. Budding yeast forms in gram stain of sputum
      C. Culture of C. albicans from bronchoscopic washings
      D. Culture of C. albicans from sputum of a patient with an abnormal
          chest X-ray
      E. None of the above
      Ref. Utz, J. P. , Buechner, H. A. : Candidosis in Management of Fungus
      Diseases of the Lung, Brechner, H. A. , (Ed), Charles C Thomas,
      Springfield, 1971, p. 179.

506. THE MOST COMMON MANIFESTATION OF BLASTOMYCOSIS WITH
      PULMONARY INVOLVEMENT IS:
      A. Weight loss
      B. Chest pain
      C. Cough
      D. Fever
      E. Hemoptysis
      Ref. Busey, J. F. : North American Blastomycosis in Management of
      Fungus Diseases of the Lungs. Buechner, H. A. , (Ed.), Charles
      C Thomas, Springfield, 1971, p. 25.

507. MOST PATIENTS WITH CRYPTOCOCCOSIS MANIFEST WHICH OF THE
      FOLLOWING DEFICIENCIES?:
      A. Deficient anticapsular antibody
      B. Myeloperoxidase deficiency
      C. Inability to phagocytose cryptococci
      D. Deficient opsonins
      E. None of the above
      Ref. Diamond, R. D. , Root, R. K. , Bennett, J. E. : Factors Influencing
      Killing of Cryptococcus Neoformans by Human Leukocytes in Vitro.
      J Inf Dis, 125:367, 1972.

508. FLUCYTOSINE IS NOT ACTIVE AGAINST:
      A. Cryptococcus neoformans
      B. Candida albicans
      C. Candida pseudotropicalis
      D. Torulopsis glabrata
      E. Coccidioides immitis
      Ref. The Medical Letter, 14:29, 1972.

509.   THE MOST COMMON FUNGI CAUSING SYSTEMIC INFECTION IN THE
        COMPROMISED HOST ARE:
        A. Candida
        B. Cryptococcus
        C. Torula
        D. Histoplasma
        E. Rhizopus
        Ref. Portnoy, J., Wolf, P. L., Webb, M.: Candida Blastospores
        and Pseudohyphae in Blood Smears. New Eng J Med, 285:1011, 1972.

510.   THE DRUG OF CHOICE FOR THE TREATMENT OF SPOROTRICHORIS
        IN CHILDREN IS:
        A. Nystatin
        B. Potassium iodide
        C. Amphotericin B
        D. Flucytosine
        E. Cytosine arabinoside
        Ref. Lynch, P., Botero, F.: Sporotrichosis in Children. Amer J Dis
        Child, 122:325, 1971.

511.   WHICH OF THE FOLLOWING DRUG REGIMENS WOULD BE EXPECTED
        TO BE THE LEAST SUCCESSFUL IN CONVERTING SPUTA OF
        TUBERCULOUS PATIENTS REQUIRING RE-TREATMENT?:
        A. Ethambutol, ethionamide
        B. Ethambutol, cycloserine, streptomycin
        C. Ethambutol
        D. Ethambutol, cycloserine
        E. Ethambutol, cycloserine, viomycin
        Ref. Pyle, M. M.: Ethambutol and Viomycin. Med Clin N Amer,
        54:1317, 1970.

512.   ALL OF THE ANTIMICROBIAL AGENTS LISTED BELOW
        ARE BACTERICIDAL FOR M. LEPRAE, EXCEPT:
        A. Dapsone
        B. Clofazimine (B663)
        C. Rifampin
        D. Ethionamide
        E. Viomycin
        Ref. Shepard, C. C., Walker, L. L., Van Landingham, R., et al:
        Kinetic Testing of Drugs Against Mycobacterium Leprae in Mice.
        Am J Trop Med Hyg, 20:616, 1971.

513.   AS PART OF A SURVEY FOR HISTOPLASMOSIS IN A NURSING HOME,
        INTRADERMAL SKIN TESTING USING HISTOPLASMIN WAS PERFORMED.
        OF THOSE REACTING NEGATIVELY, WHAT PERCENT WOULD BE
        EXPECTED TO BE CONVERTED TO POSITIVE BY ANOTHER
        HISTOPLASMIN SKIN TEST 3 WEEKS LATER?:
        A. 35%
        B. 0%
        C. 1%
        D. Less than 10%
        E. 75%
        Ref. Ganley, J. P., Smith, R. E., Thomas, D. B., et al: Booster
        Effect of Histoplasmin Skin Testing in an Elderly Population. Amer J
        Epidem, 95:104, 1972.

514. ALL OF THE FOLLOWING ARE CHARACTERISTICS OF ALLERGIC
BRONCHOPULMONARY ASPERGILLOSIS, EXCEPT:
A. Peripheral eosinophilia
B. Positive immediate skin responses to Aspergillus
C. Presence of serum precipitins to Aspergillus extract
D. Pulmonary infiltrate
E. Poor response to corticosteroid therapy
Ref. Jordan, M. C. , Bierman, W. , van Arsdel, P. P. , Jr.: Allergic
Bronchopulmonary Aspergillosis. Arch Intern Med, 128:577, 1971.

515. THE MOST COMMON MANIFESTATION OF PRIMARY INFECTION
WITH COCCIDIOIDES IMMITIS IS:
A. Erythema nodosum
B. Influenza-like syndrome
C. No clinical manifestations
D. Meningitis
E. Pneumonia
Ref. Smith, J. W.: Coccidioidomycosis. Texas Med, 67:117, 1971.

516. THE CHARACTERISTIC LESION OF CANDIDA ENDOPHTHALMITIS IS:
A. Roth spot
B. Angioid streak
C. Round white lesion with pre-retinal haze
D. Optic atrophy
E. Anterior uveitis
Ref. Fishman, L. S. , Griffin, J. R. , Sapico, F. L. , et al: Hematogeneous
Candida Endophthalmitis - A Complication of Candidemia. New Eng J Med,
286:675, 1972.

517. THE HEMATOLOGIC MANIFESTATION MOST COMMONLY
ENCOUNTERED IN PROGRESSIVE DISSEMINATED HISTOPLASMOSIS IS:
A. Leukocytosis
B. Leukopenia
C. Splenomegaly
D. Positive bone marrow culture
E. Anemia
Ref. Smith, J. W. , Utz, J. P.: Progressive Disseminated Histoplasmosis.
Ann Intern Med, 76:557, 1972.

518. WHICH OF THE FOLLOWING IS LEAST LIKELY TO YIELD A POSITIVE
CULTURE FOR HISTOPLASMA CAPSULATUM IN PROGRESSIVE
DISSEMINATED HISTOPLASMOSIS?:
A. Oral ulcers
B. Lymph nodes
C. Bone marrow
D. Livery biopsy
E. Urine
Ref. Smith, J. W. , Utz, J. P.: Progressive Disseminated Histoplasmosis.
Ann Intern Med, 76:557, 1972.

519. WHICH OF THE FOLLOWING TESTS IS MOST LIKELY TO REVEAL
ANTIBODIES TO ASPERIGILLUS FUMIGATUS IN PATIENTS WITH
WIDESPREAD INVASIVE ASPERGILLOSIS?:
A. Double diffusion in agar
B. Complement fixation
C. Immunoelectrophoresis
D. Indirect fluorescent antibody
E. None of the above
Ref. Young, R. C. , Bennett, J. E.: Invasive Aspergillosis: Absence
of Detectable Antibody. Am Rev Resp Dis, 104:710, 1971.

520.   OPHTHALMIC COCCIDIOIDOMYCOSIS PRODUCES:
   A. Corneal ulcers
   B. Retinal vein thrombosis
   C. Hypopon
   D. Choroidal granulomata
   E. Conjunctivitis
   Ref. Olavarria, R., Fajardo, L. F.: Ophthalmic Coccidioidomycosis.
   Arch Path, 92:191, 1971.

521.   A RISING AGGLUTINATING OR PRECIPITATING ANTIBODY TITER
   AGAINST CANDIDA sp. DURING ACUTE LEUKEMIA IS MOST LIKELY TO
   BE ASSOCIATED WITH:
   A. Tuberculosis
   B. Spontaneous fever
   C. Visceral candidiasis
   D. Non-candida mycotic disease
   E. None of the above
   Ref. Preisler, H. D., Hasenclever, H. F., Henderson, E. S.: Anti-
   Candida Antibodies in Patients with Leukemia: Prospective Study.
   Am J Med, 51:352, 1971.

522.   WHICH OF THE FOLLOWING DRUGS IS THE LEAST TOXIC AND MOST
   EFFECTIVE AGENT FOR TREATMENT OF SPOROTRICHOSIS?:
   A. Amphotericin B
   B. Cyclophosphamide
   C. Erythromycin
   D. Hydroxystilbamidine
   E. Potassium iodide
   Ref. Orr, E. R., Riley, H. D.: Sporotrichosis in Childhood: Report
   of Ten Cases. J Pediat, 78:951, 1971.

523.   THE FOLLOWING DIAGRAM ILLUSTRATES A CONCEPT OF THE
   RELATIONSHIP OF THE CELLS INVOLVED IN THE PRODUCTION OF
   THE TUBERCULOSIS GRANULOMA:

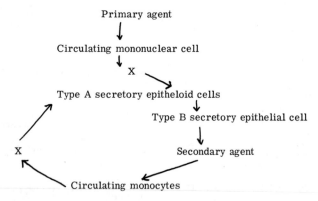

IDENTIFY "X" FROM THE FOLLOWING LIST:
   A. Polymorphonuclear leukocyte
   B. Mast cells
   C. Stimulated mononuclear cell
   D. Downey cell
   E. M. tuberculosis
   Ref. Williams, W. J., Erasmus, D. A., Valerie-James, E. M., et al:
   The Fine Structure of Sarcoid and Tuberculous Granulomas.
   Postgrad Med J, 46:496, 1970.

THE FOLLOWING QUESTIONS CONSIST OF PAIRS OF PHRASES
DESCRIBING CONDITIONS OR QUANTITIES WHICH MAY OR MAY NOT
VARY IN RELATION TO EACH OTHER. ANSWER:
A. If increase in the first is accompanied by increase in the second or
    decrease in the first is accompanied by decrease in the second
B. If increase in the first is accompanied by decrease in the second or
    decrease in the first is accompanied by increase in the second
C. If changes in the first are independent of changes in the second

524. 1. Use of rifampin in treatment of chronic non-tuberculous broncho-
          pulmonary infections
      2. Resistance of H. influenzae, isolated from rifampin treated patients
          to rifampin
      Ref. Citron, K. M. , May, J. R. : Rifamycin Antibiotics in Chronic
      Purulent Bronchitis. Lancet, 2:982, 1969.

525. 1. Age
      2. Dermal hypersensitivity to tuberculin
      Ref. Woodruff, C. E. , Chapman, P. T. : Tuberculin Sensitivity in Elderly
      Patients. Am Rev Resp Dis, 104:261, 1971.

526. 1. Titer of serum complement fixing antibody against histoplasmal
          antigens
      2. Lymphocyte transformation using histoplasmal antigens
      Ref. Alford, R. H. , Goodwin, R. A. : Patterns of Immune Response in
      Chronic Pulmonary Histoplasmosis. J Infect Dis, 125:269, 1972.

527. 1. Growth of C. albicans in vitro during 18 hours
      2. Number of acid phosphatase positive particles per cell
      Ref. Montes, L. F. , Wilborn, W. H. : Acid Phosphatase Activity During
      Phases of Growth in Candida Albicans. Int J Derm, 9:220, 1970.

528. 1. Concentration of glucose in saliva
      2. Growth of C. albicans in saliva
      Ref. Knight, L. , Fletcher, J. : Growth of Candida Albicans in Saliva.
      J Infect Dis, 123:371, 1971.

529. 1. Length of time patient has had chronic pulmonary histoplasmosis
      2. Skin reactivity to histoplasmin
      Ref. Alford, R. H. , Goodwin, R. A. : Patterns of Immune Response in
      Chronic Pulmonary Histoplasmosis. J Infec Dis, 125:269, 1972.

THE FOLLOWING QUESTIONS CONSIST OF A STATEMENT AND A
REASON. SELECT:
A. If both statement and reason are true and the reason is the correct
    explanation of the statement
B. If both statement and reason are true but the reason is not the correct
    explanation of the statement
C. If the statement is true but the reason is false
D. If the statement is false but the reason is true
E. If both statement and reason are false

530. ___ Coccidioidin skin tests are of prognostic value in disseminated
          coccidioidomycosis BECAUSE patients with disseminated coccidioi-
          domycosis frequently show very marked delayed hypersensitivity
          responses to coccidioidin.
      Ref. Werner, S. B. , Pappagianis, D. , Heindl, I. , et al: An Epidemic
      of Coccidioidomycosis Among Archeology Students in Northern
      California. New Eng J Med, 286:507, 1972.

531. ___ In the complement fixation antibody test for histoplasmosis, both a soluble mycelial filtrate (histoplasmin) and a suspension of intact yeast cells of H. capsulatum are used as antigens BECAUSE sera from culturally proven cases of histoplasmosis may react to only one of the antigens.
Ref. Kaufman, L.: Serology: Its Value in the Diagnosis of Coccidioidomycosis, Cryptococcosis, and Histoplasmosis. Proc Int Symp on Mycoses, Pan American Health Organization, Washington, D.C., 1970, pp. 96-100.

532. ___ Blood for histoplasmin serology should be obtained prior to skin testing with histoplasmin BECAUSE 10-15% of histoplasmin sensitive persons may produce both complement fixing and precipitin antibodies in response to a single histoplasmin test.
Ref. Kaufman, L.: Serology: Its Value in the Diagnosis of Coccidioidomycosis, Cryptococcis, and Histoplasmosis. Proc Int Symp on Mycoses, Pan American Health Organization, Washington, D.C., pp. 96-100.

533. ___ Tuberculin hypersensitivity probably does not play a large role in acquired immunity to tuberculosis BECAUSE immunity to tuberculous infection can be produced without concomitant tuberculin hypersensitivity.
Ref. Youmans, G.P.: The Role of Lymphocytes and Other Factors in Antimicrobial Cellular Immunity. J Reticuloendoth Soc., 10:100, 1971.

534. ___ Candida paropsilosis is less virulent than Candida albicans BECAUSE C. paropsilosis is unable to transform into the mycelial phase in tissue.
Ref. Goldstein, E., Hoeprich, P.D.; Problems in the Diagnosis and Treatment of Systemic Candidiasis. J Infect Dis, 125:190, 1972.

535. ___ BCG vaccination is consistently protective against leprosy BECAUSE cross protection is known to exist between BCG vaccine and infections with mycobacteria other than M. tuberculosis.
Ref. Rees, R.J.W., Waters, M.F.R.: Recent Trends in Leprosy Research. Brit Med Bull, 28:16, 1972.

536. ___ Annual tuberculin testing for general hospital employees should continue BECAUSE the greatest risk of new tuberculous infection arises from individuals with unrecognized or untreated open disease.
Ref. Atuk, N.O., Hunt, R.N.: Serial Tuberculin Testing and Isoniazid Therapy in General Hospital Employees. JAMA, 218:1795, 1971.

ANSWER THE FOLLOWING QUESTIONS ACCORDING TO THE KEY BELOW:
A. If choice A is greater than choice B
B. If choice B is greater than choice A
C. If A and B are equal or nearly equal

537. GROWTH OF CANDIDA SPECIES ON MEDIA CONTAINING:
A. No gentamicin
B. Gentamicin 5 mcg/ml
Ref. Dolan, C.T.: Effect of Gentamicin on Growth of Yeasts, Yeast-Like Organisms, and Asperigillus Fumigatus. Amer J Clin Path, 57:30, 1972.

538. PROBABILITY OF IDENTIFYING SPOROTRICHUM BY:
A. Gram stain of exudate from lesion
B. Culture of the lesion
Ref. Park, C. H. , Greer, C. L. , Cook, C. B. : Cutaneous Sporotrichosis.
AJCP, 57:23, 1972.

539. IN PROGRESSIVE DISSEMINATED HISTOPLASMOSIS, WHICH OCCURS
MOST FREQUENTLY?:
A. Pulmonary infiltrates
B. Hepatocellular functional abnormalities
Ref. Smith, J. W. , Utz, J. P. : Progressive Disseminated Histoplasmosis.
Ann Intern Med, 76:557, 1972.

540. WHICH OF THE FOLLOWING IS MOST SPECIFIC IN THE DIAGNOSIS OF
SYSTEMIC CANDIDIASIS?:
A. Serum precipitating antibody against cytoplasmic candida antigens
B. Serum candida agglutinating antibody
Ref. Taschdjian, C. L. , Kozinn, P. J. , Cuesta, M. B. , Toni, E. F. :
Serodiagnosis of Candidal Infections. Amer J Clin Path, 57:195, 1972.

541. AMOUNT OF ADMINISTERED DOSE OF:
A. Amphotericin B excreted in urine
B. Flucytosine (5-FC) excreted in urine
Ref. Utz, J. P. : Flucytosine. New Eng J Med, 286:114, 1972.

542. NUMBERS OF PERSONS WITH POSITIVE HISTOPLASMIN SKIN TESTS
WHO ARE:
A. Normal controls
B. Patients with ocular histoplasmosis
Ref. Smith, R. E. , Ganley, J. P. : Presumed Ocular Histoplasmosis:
I: Histoplasmin Skin Test Sensitivity in Cases identified During a
Community Survey. Arch Ophthalmol, 87:245, 1972.

543. WHICH OF THESE SEROLOGIC TESTS USING AN ULTRASONIC
ANTIGEN IS MORE SPECIFIC FOR EXTRACUTANEOUS SPOROTRICHOSIS?:
A. Complement fixing antigen
B. Precipitation test
Ref. Roberts, G. D. , Larsh, H. W. : The Serologic Diagnosis of
Extracutaneous Sporotrichosis. Amer J Clin Path, 56:597, 1971.

544. THE FREQUENCY OF "M-TYPE" GLOBULINEMIA IN THE SERA OF:
A. Tuberculous patients
B. Population at large
Ref. Chung, D. K. : Frequency of "M-Type" Globulinemia Among a
Tuberculosis Hospital Population. Chest, 60:537, 1971.

545. SERUM ANTIBODY (PRECIPITINS OR COMPLEMENT FIXING
ANTIBODY) AGAINST A. FUMIGATUS IN PATIENTS WITH:
A. Widespread invasive aspergillosis
B. Bronchopulmonary aspergillosis
Ref. Young, R. C. , Bennett, J. E. : Invasive Aspergillosis. Am Rev
Resp Dis, 104:710, 1971.

546. PATIENTS WITH TUBERCULOUS PERITONITIS WHO HAVE:
A. Bloody ascitic fluid
B. Non-bloody ascitic fluid
Ref. Borhanmanesh, F. , Hekmat, K. , Vaezzadah, K. , et al:
Tuberculous Peritonitis. Ann Intern Med, 76:567, 1972.

547.   RESISTANCE TO REINFECTION WITH C. IMMITIS OF MICE IMMUNIZED:
        A. Intravenously with C. immitis spherules
        B. By the intramuscular injection of C. immitis spherules
        Ref. Levine, H. B. , Scalarone, G. M.: Deficient Resistance to
        Coccidioides Immitis Following Intravenous Vaccination. Saboraudia,
        9:81, 1971, Ibid, 9:90, Ibid, 9:97.

548.   FIVE YEAR SURVIVAL RATE:
        A. Without therapy for blastomycosis
        B. After therapy for blastomycosis
        Ref. Furcolow, M. L. , Watson, K. T. , Tisdall, O. F. , et al: Some
        Factors Affecting Survival in Systemic Blastomycosis. Dis Chest,
        54:285, 1968.

549.   PERCENTAGE OF:
        A. Pleural fluid obtained from idiopathic effusions which are culturally
            positive for M. tuberculosis
        B. Pleural biopsies from idiopathic effusions which are culturally
            positive for M. tuberculosis
        Ref. Scerbo, J. , Keltz, H. , Stone, D. J. : A Prospective Study of
        Closed Pleural Biopsies. JAMA, 218:377, 1971.

550.   RISK OF DEVELOPING:
        A. Active pulmonary tuberculosis in household contacts for 1 year after
            diagnosis of index case of active pulmonary tuberculosis
        B. Liver disease for household contacts receiving INH during 1 year
            after diagnosis of index cases of active pulmonary tuberculosis
        Ref. Meade, G. M. : Isoniazid and the Liver: FDA Drug Bulletin
        October, 1971, p. 3.

551.   A. Minimum inhibiting concentration of clotrimazole (Bay b 5097)
            for blastomyces dermatitidis, histoplasma capsulatum and
            coccidioides immitis
        B. Minimum inhibitory concentration of amphotericin B for the same
            organisms listed in A (above)
        Ref. Shadomy, S.: In Vitro Activity of Clotrimazole, (Bay b 5097).
        Inf and Imm, 4:143, 1971.

552.   PERCENTAGE OF UNTREATED TUBERCULOUS PATIENTS WHOSE:
        A. Pleural fluid is positive for M. tuberculosis by culture
        B. Pleural biopsy is positive for M tuberculosis by culture
        Ref. Scerbo, J. , Keltz, H. , Stone, D. J. : A Prospective Study of
        Closed Pleural Biopsies. JAMA, 218:377, 1971.

553.   SENSITIVITY OF:
        A. Cryptococcus neoformans to amphotericin B
        B. Coccidioides immitis to amphotericin B
        Ref. Seabury, J. H.: The Treatment of Coccidioidomycosis, Cryptococcosis
        and Histoplasmosis. Proc Int Symp on Mycoses, Pan American Health
        Organization, Washington, D. C. , 1970, pp. 128-134.

554.   CLINICAL CASES OF:
        A. Blastomycosis per year in the United States
        B. Histoplasmosis per year in the United States
        Ref. Ajello, L. : The Medical Mycological Iceberg. Proc Int Symp on
        Mycoses, Pan American Health Organization, Washington, D. C. , 1970,
        pp. 3-12.

555. CLINICAL CASES OF:
A. Cryptococcosis per year in the United States
B. Coccidioidomycosis per year in the United States
Ref. Ajello, L.: The Medical Mycological Iceberg. Proc Int Symp on Mycoses, Pan American Health Organization, Washington, D.C., 1970, pp. 3-12.

556. RESISTANCE OF:
A. Group I atypical mycobacteria to rifampin
B. Group III atypical mycobacteria to rifampin
Ref. Rynearson, T.K., Shronts, J.S., Wolinsky, E.: Rifampin: In Vitro Effect on Atypical Mycobacteria. Am Rev Resp Dis, 104:272-274, 1971.

EACH SET OF LETTERED HEADINGS IS FOLLOWED BY A NUMBERED LIST OF WORDS OR PHRASES. ANSWER:
A. If the word or phrase is associated with A only
B. If the word or phrase is associated with B only
C. If the word or phrase is associated with A and B
D. If the word or phrase is associated with neither A nor B

A. Photochromogens
B. Scotochromogens
C. Both
D. Neither

557. ___ Runyon Group III
558. ___ M. Kansasii
559. ___ Gause bacillus
560. ___ Yellow pigment in light or dark
561. ___ M fortuitum
562. ___ Battey bacillus
Ref. Freedsom, S.O.: Tuberculin Testing and Screening: A Critical Evaluation. Hospital Practice, 7:63, 1972.

A. Serum clumping factor for C. albicans
B. Serum factor interfering with action of C. albicans clumping factor
C. Both
D. Neither

563. ___ Present in most healthy adult serum
564. ___ Reduced in azotemia and diabetic acidosis
565. ___ Antibody elicited by candida
566. ___ Macroeuglobulin
Ref. Smith, J.K., Louria, D.B., Anti-Candida Factors in Serum and Their Inhibitors. II. Identification of a Candida-Clumping Factor and the Influence of the Immune Response on the Morphology of Candida and on Anti-Candida Activity of Serum in Rabbits. J Infect Dis, 125:115, 1972.

A. Actinomycosis
B. Nocardiosis
C. Both
D. Neither

567. ___ Amphotericin B drug of choice for treatment
568. ___ Penicillin
569. ___ Sulfonamides
570. ___ Hyphae with true branching
        Ref. Seabury, J. H.: Actinomycosis and Nocardiosis in Management of
        Fungus Disease of the Lungs, Buechner, H. A., (ed), Charles C Thomas,
        Springfield, 1971, p. 197.

A. Tuberculosis
B. Coccidioidomycosis
C. Both
D. Neither

571. ___ Infiltrative lesions in upper lobes of lung
572. ___ Pleural effusion
573. ___ Pulmonary cavities
574. ___ Solid granulomata in lung
        Ref. Einstein, H. A.: Coccidioidomycosis in Management of Fungus
        Diseases of the Lung, Buechner, H. A., (ed), Charles C Thomas,
        Springfield, 1971, p. 124.

A. Tuberculosis
B. Histoplasmosis
C. Both
D. Neither

575. ___ Usually present in upper lobes
576. ___ Calcification and fibrosis common
577. ___ Skin test may be negative with acute dissemination
578. ___ Complement fixation test useful in diagnosis
        Ref. Wagley, P. F., Johns, C. J., Cader, G., et al: Bronchopulmonary
        Suppuration, Chap. 40 in The Principles and Practice of Medicine, 17th
        Ed Appleton-Century-Crofts, New York, 1968, pp. 402-410.

A. Productive cough
B. Non-productive cough
C. Both
D. Neither

579. ___ Tuberculosis
580. ___ Mycoplasma pneumonia
581. ___ Bronchiectasis
582. ___ Typhoid fever
583. ___ Varicella
584. ___ Coccidioidomycosis
585. ___ Tetanus
        Ref. Fekety, F. R., Cluff, L. E.: The Clinical and Laboratory
        Manifestations of Infectious Diseases in The Principles and Practice
        of Medicine. 17th Ed, Chap 66, Appleton-Century-Crofts, New York,
        1968, pp. 654-671.

IN THE FOLLOWING QUESTIONS, CHOOSE:
A. If 1, 2 and 3 are correct
B. If 1 and 3 are correct
C. If 2 and 4 are correct
D. If only 4 is correct
E. If all four are correct

586. MASS CHEST X-RAY SCREENING IS NO LONGER JUSTIFIED FOR
DETECTION OF NEW CASES OF TUBERCULOSIS. WHICH OF THE
FOLLOWING GROUPS WOULD JUSTIFIABLY BE SURVEYED ANNUALLY
BY SELECTIVE CHEST RADIOGRAPHY?:
1. School teachers
2. Hospital employees
3. Food handlers
4. Transportation workers
Ref. Freedman, S. O.: Tuberculin Testing and Screening: A Critical
Evaluation. Hospital Practice, 7:63, 1972.

587. FLUCYTOSINE IS ACTIVE AGAINST:
1. H. capsulatum
2. C. immitis
3. B. dermatitidis
4. C. albicans
Ref. The Medical Letter, 14:29, 1972.

588. WHICH OF THE FOLLOWING FACTORS ARE RESPONSIBLE FOR THE
ANEMIA SEEN IN ACTIVE PULMONARY TUBERCULOSIS BEFORE
CHEMOTHERAPY?:
1. Defective iron utilization
2. Iron deficiency
3. Folate deficiency
4. Vitamin B_{12} deficiency
Ref. Line, D. H., Seitanidis, B., Morgan, J. O., et al: The Effects of
Chemotherapy on Iron, Folate and Vitamin B_{12} Metabolism in Tuberculosis. Quart J Med, 40:331, 1971.

589. WHICH OF THE FOLLOWING ARE COMPLICATIONS OF TUBERCULOSIS
MASTOIDITIS?:
1. Facial paralysis
2. Postauricular fistula
3. Hearing loss
4. Proptosis
Ref. Wolfowitz, B. L.: Tuberculous Mastoiditis. Arch Otolaryngol,
95:109, 1972.

590. IN MICE, THE EFFECT OF DAPSONE ON MYCOBACTERIUM LEPRAE
IS TO:
1. Induce resistance to dapsone
2. Kill mycobacterium
3. Excite host response to the organism
4. Prolong the lag phase of multiplication
Ref. Levy, L.: Prolongation of the Lag Phase of Mycobacterium Leprae
by Dapsone. Proc Soc Expl Biol Med, 139:263, 1972.

591. TUBERCULOSIS OF THE FEMALE GENITAL TRACT IS MOST OFTEN
      ASSOCIATED WITH:
      1. Abdominal swelling
      2. Dysmenorrhea
      3. Vaginal discharge
      4. Infertility
      Ref. Ojo, O. A., Onifade, A., Akande, E. O.: The Pattern of Female
      Genital Tuberculosis in Ibadan. Israel J Med Sci, 7:280, 1971.

592. THE SKIN MANIFESTATIONS OF PRIMARY COCCIDIOIDOMYCOSIS
      INCLUDE:
      1. Erythema nodosum
      2. Generalized maculopapular eruption
      3. Erythema multiforme
      4. Urticaria
      Ref. Werner, S. B., Pappagianis, D., Heindl, I., et al: An Epidemic of
      Coccidioidomycosis Among Archeology Students in Northern California.
      New Eng J Med, 286:507, 1972.

593. TUBERCULOUS OTITIS MEDIA IS CHARACTERIZED BY:
      1. Most patients are children less than 1 year of age
      2. Strongly positive PPD intradermal test
      3. Profound hearing loss
      4. Absence of associated pulmonary lesion
      Ref. Saltzman, S. J., Feigin, R. D.: Tuberculous Otitis Media and
      Mastoiditis. J Pediat, 79:1004, 1971.

594. WHICH OF THE FOLLOWING HAVE BEEN INCRIMINATED IN THE
      ETIOLOGY OF M. FORTUITUM INFECTIONS ?:
      1. Lawn mower injuries
      2. Injections of drugs
      3. Gunshot wounds
      4. Foreign body corneal injuries
      Ref. Offer, R. C., Karlson, A. G., Spittell, J. A.: Infection Caused
      by Mycobacterium Fortuitum. Mayo Clin Proc, 46:747, 1971.

595. WHICH OF THE FOLLOWING PERMIT MOST ACCURATE IDENTIFICATION
      OF VISCERAL CANDIDIOSIS AFFECTING PATIENTS WITH LEUKEMIA?:
      1. Blood cultures positive for C.albicans
      2. Fever unresponsive to antibiotic therapy
      3. Rising serum agglutinating antibody to C.albicans
      4. Presence of gastrointestinal candidiosis
      Ref. Preisler, H. D., Hasenclever, H. F., Henderson, E. S.: Anti-
      Candida Antibodies in Patients with Acute Leukemia. Amer J Med,
      51:352, 1971.

596. ASPERGILLOMAS MAY OCCUR IN PULMONARY CAVITIES CAUSED BY
      THE FOLLOWING DISEASES:
      1. Sarcoid
      2. Tuberculosis
      3. Carcinoma
      4. Blastomycosis
      Ref. Sarosi, G. A., Silberfarb, P. M., Saliba, N. A., et al: Aspergillomas
      Occuring in Blastomycotic Cavities. Amer Rev Resp Dis, 104:581, 1971.

597. WHICH OF THE FOLLOWING ARE THOUGHT TO BE INVOLVED IN THE
      PATHOGENESIS OF DISSEMINATED CANDIDIASIS?:
      1. Myeloperoxidase deficiency of granulocytes
      2. Antimicrobial therapy
      3. Prolonged use of intravenous catheters
      4. Adrenocorticosteroid therapy
      Ref. Quie, P. G. , Chilgren, R. A. : Acute Disseminated and Chronic
      Mucocutaneous Candidiosis. Seminars in Hematology, 8:227, 1971.

598. THE FOLLOWING ARE CHARACTERISTICS OF CHRONIC MUCO-
      CUTANEOUS CANDIDIOSIS:
      1. Follows prolonged use of intravenous catheters
      2. Association with endocrinopathies
      3. Generalized cutaneous hyperergy
      4. Complement fixing antibodies against candida sp. usually elevated
      Ref. Quie, P. G. , Chilgren, R. A. : Acute Disseminated and Chronic
      Mucocutaneous Candidiosis. Seminars in Hematology, 8:227, 1971.

599. ASPERIGILLUS INFECTION SHOULD BE CONSIDERED WHEN A
      PATIENT RECEIVING STEROIDS OR ANTIBIOTICS DEVELOPS:
      1. Microangiopathic hemolytic anemia
      2. Leukoerythroblastosis
      3. Disseminated intravascular coagulation
      4. Petechiae
      Ref. Rabboy, S. J. , Salisbury, K. , Ragsdale, B. , et al: Mechanism of
      Aspergillus Induced Microangiopathic Hemolytic Anemia. Arch Intern
      Med, 128:790, 1971.

600. WHICH OF THE FOLLOWING CHARACTERISTICS OF PATIENTS WITH
      BLASTOMYCOSIS WOULD LEAD TO TREATMENT WITH AMPHOTERICIN
      B RATHER THAN HYDROXYSTILBAMIDINE ISETHIONATE?:
      1. Patient with cavitary pulmonary blastomycosis
      2. Patient with pre-existing renal failure
      3. Patient with blastomycosis involving the liver as well as the lung
      4. Patient with blastomycosis of the skin without any pulmonary disease
      Ref. Busey, J. F. : North American Blastomycosis in Management of
      Fungus Diseases of the Lung. Buechner, H. A. , (ed), Charles C Thomas,
      Springfield, 1971, pp. 47-48.

601. THE FOLLOWING SIGNS ARE FOUND IN MORE THAN HALF OF THOSE
      PATIENTS WITH DISSEMINATED HISTOPLASMOSIS:
      1. Meningitis
      2. Fever
      3. Hypotension (blood pressure less than 90 mm Hg syst)
      4. Hepatosplenomegaly
      Ref. Sarosi, G. A. , Voth, D. W. , Dahl, B. A. , et al: Disseminated
      Histoplasmosis: Results of Long-Term Follow-Up. Ann Intern Med,
      75:511-516, 1971.

602. IN REFERENCE TO SEROLOGY FOLLOWING PRIMARY COCCIDIOIDO-
      MYCOSIS, WHICH OF THE FOLLOWING STATEMENTS ARE ACCURATE?:
      1. The complement fixing antibody titers parallel the severity of the
          infection
      2. The precipitating antibody test is most effective in detecting early cases
      3. Precipitating antibody titers are seldom detected 6 months after
          infection
      4. Positive serological results are seldom accompanied by a positive
          coccidioidin skin test
      Ref. Kaufman, L. : Serology: Its Value in the Diagnosis of Coccidioido-
      mycosis, Cryptococcosis, and Histoplasmosis. Proc Int Symp on Mycoses.
      Pan American Health Organization, Washington, D. C. , 1970, pp. 96-100.

603. WHICH OF THE FOLLOWING MICROORGANISMS ARE INHIBITED BY
     CONCENTRATIONS OF 5 FLUOROCYTOSINE WHICH CAN BE OBTAINED
     USING RECOMMENDED ORAL DOSE REGIMENS OF 100 TO 150 mg/kgl/
     DAY?:
     1. C. albicans
     2. C. neoformans
     3. T. glabrata
     4. Aspergillus sp.
     Ref. Steer, P. L., Marks, M. I., Klite, P. D., et al: 5-Fluorocytosine:
     An Oral Antifungal Compound. Ann Int Med, 76:15, 1972.

604. ATYPICAL MYCOBACTERIA OF RUNYON GROUP II (SCOTOCHROMO-
     GENS) HAVE BEEN REPORTED TO PRODUCE TUBERCULOSIS-LIKE
     DISEASE IN THE FOLLOWING ORGANS OR WITH THE FOLLOWING
     CHARACTERISTICS:
     1. Lung
     2. Lymph nodes (adenitis)
     3. Kidneys
     4. Disseminated miliary disease
     Ref. McNutt, D. R., Fudenberg, H. H.: Disseminated Scotochromogen
     Infection and Unusual Myeloproliferative Disorder. Ann Intern Med,
     75:737, 1971.

605. WHICH OF THE FOLLOWING STATEMENTS CONCERNING TUBER-
     CULOSIS OF THE BREAST ARE CORRECT?:
     1. Axillary tuberculous lumph adenopathy on the involved side is very
        common
     2. Pulmonary tuberculosis is almost never coexistent
     3. Most cases occur in patients 20 to 50 years of age
     4. Can be separated from carcinoma of the breast by mammography
     Ref. Murkerjee, P., Cohen, R. V., Niden, A. H.: Tuberculosis of
     the Breast. Am Rev Resp Dis, 104:661, 1971.

     EACH GROUP OF ITEMS CONSISTS OF A LIST OF LETTERED HEADINGS
     FOLLOWED BY A LIST OF NUMBERED WORDS OR PHRASES. FOR
     EACH NUMBERED WORD OR PHRASE, SELECT THE ONE HEADING
     MOST CLOSELY RELATED TO IT:

     A. Anergy to PPD
     B. Absorption of PPD
     C. Inadequate dose of antigen
     D. Instability of PPD

606. ___ Jet gun injectors
607. ___ Tween-80
608. ___ Rubeola
609. ___ Immunosupressive drugs
610. ___ PPD tablets
     Ref. Edwards, P. Q.: Tuberculin Negative? New Eng J Med, 286:373,
     1972.

A. Hamycin
B. 5-flurocytosine
C. Clotrimazole

611. ___ Blastomycosis
612. ___ Dermatophytic infection
613. ___ Candidiasis
614. ___ Cryptococcosis
Ref. Shadomy, S.: What's New in Antifungal Chemotherapy. Clin Med, 79:14, 1972.

A. Tuberculosis
B. Amebic abscess
C. Aspergillosis
D. Actinomycosis
E. Bronchogenic carcinoma

615. ___ Sputum almost invariably positive in untreated cases
616. ___ Mycetoma
617. ___ Therapeutic response to emitine
618. ___ Chest wall sinuses
619. ___ May occur in pulmonary segments not often affected by aspiration
Ref. Wagley, P. F., Johns, C. J., Cader, G., et al: Bronchopulmonary Suppuration, Chap 40 in The Principles and Practice of Medicine, 17th Ed, Appleton-Century-Crofts, New York, 1968, pp. 402-410.

A. Osseous coccidioidomycosis
B. Osseous tuberculosis
C. Osseous actinomycosis
D. Bacterial osteomyelitis

620. ___ Destruction of more than one joint common; weight-bearing portion of joint usually spared
621. ___ Involvement of mandible and facial bones
622. ___ Multiple lesions in bony prominences and metaphyses
623. ___ Joint destruction and early periosteal new bone formation
Ref. Dalinka, M. K., Dinnenberg, S., Greendyke, W. H., et al: Roentgenographic Features of Osseous Coccidioidomycosis and Differential Diagnosis. J Bone Joint Surg, 53:1157, 1971.

FOR EACH OF THE FOLLOWING MULTIPLE CHOICE QUESTIONS,
SELECT THE ONE MOST APPROPRIATE ANSWER:

624.   THE LOWEST CONCENTRATION OF PENICILLIN G WHICH EXCEEDS
        THE MIC FOR GREATER THAN 80% OF STRAINS OF FUSOBACTERIUM,
        CLOSTRIDIUM, AND PEPTOCOCCUS sp. IS (IN UG/ML):
        A. 0.05   D. 6.2
        B. 0.2   E. 25
        C. 0.8
        Ref. Martin, W. J., Gardner, M., Washington, J. A.: In Vitro Anti-
        microbial Susceptibility of Anaerobic Bacteria Isolated from Clinical
        Specimens. Antimicrob Ag Chemother, 1:148, 1972.

625.   WHICH OF THE FOLLOWING ANTIBIOTICS IS THE BEST CHOICE IN
        TREATING SERRATIA MARCESCENS BACTEREMIA?:
        A. Kanamycin   D. Gentamicin
        B. Cephalothin   E. Carbenicillin
        C. Chloramphenicol
        Ref. Crowder, J. G., Gilkey, G. H., White, A. C.: Serratia Marcescens
        Bacteremia. Arch Intern Med, 128:247, 1971.

626.   ALL OF THE FOLLOWING ANTIBIOTIC REGIMENS ARE ACCEPTABLE
        FOR THE TREATMENT OF GONORRHEA IN THE MALE, EXCEPT:
        A. Aqueous procaine penicillin
        B. Oral phenoxymethyl penicillin
        C. Ampicillin with probenecid
        D. Tetracycline
        Ref. Kvale, P. A., Keys, T. F., Johnson, D. W., Holmes, K. K.:
        Single Oral Dose Ampicillin-Probenecid Treatment of Gonorrhea in the
        Male. JAMA, 215:1449, 1971.

627.   CHOOSE THE ANTIMICROBIC TO WHICH MOST STRAINS OF SERRATIA
        SPECIES (ISOLATED FROM SPUTUM AND URINE) WOULD BE
        SENSITIVE:
        A. Ampicillin   D. Colistin
        B. Cephalothin   E. Gentamicin
        C. Nitrofurantoin
        Ref. Crowder, J. G., Gilkey, G. H., White, A. C.: Serratia Marcescens
        Bacteremia. Arch Int Med, 128:247, 1971.

628.   WHICH OF THE FOLLOWING TOPICAL ANTIBIOTICS IS CONSISTENTLY
        EFFECTIVE IN ERADICATING BACTERIA FROM THE EYELID PRIOR
        TO OPHTHALMIC SURGERY?:
        A. Gentamicin   D. Chloramphenicol
        B. Neomycin   E. None of the above
        C. Polymycin
        Ref. Whitney, C. R., Andersen, R. P., Allansmith, M. R.: Pre-
        operatively Administered Antibiotics. Arch Ophthalmol, 87:155, 1972.

629.   THE DRUG OF FIRST CHOICE FOR TREATMENT OF MOST URINARY
        TRACT INFECTIONS IN DOMICILIARY PRACTICE IS:
        A. A sulfonamide   D. Tetracycline
        B. Nalidixic acid   E. Nitrofurantoin
        C. Ampicillin
        Ref. Harvey, K. J., Smith, D. D.: Antimicrobial Sensitivity Patterns
        as a Guide to Domiciliary Treatment of Urinary Tract Infections.
        Med J Aust, 1:177, 1972.

630. WHICH OF THE FOLLOWING CEPHALOSPORIN DERIVATIVES IS
     GENERALLY MORE ACTIVE AGAINST GRAM-POSITIVE BACTERIA
     THAN THE OTHERS IN VITRO?:
     A. Cephalexin   D. Cephaloglycin
     B. Cephalothin   E. Desacetylcephaloglycin
     C. Cephaloridine
     Ref. Kayser, F. H.: In Vitro Activity of Cephalosporin Antibiotics
     Against Gram Positive Bacteria. Postgrad Med J, 47:14, 1971.

631. THE PERCENTAGE OF FECAL FLORA WHICH BECOME RESISTANT
     TO AN ORALLY ABSORBABLE ANTIBIOTIC AFTER USE OF THE
     ORALLY ABSORBABLE ANTIBIOTIC IS:
     A. 5   D. 20
     B. 0.1   E. 99
     C. 75
     Ref. Bodey, G. P.: Oral Antibiotic Prophylaxis in Protected Environ-
     ment Units: Effect of Nonabsorbable and Absorbable Antibiotics on the
     Fecal Flora. Antimicrob Ag Chemother, 1:343, 1972.

632. THE SINGLE MOST COMMON CAUSE OF DEATH IN CRITICAL CARE
     UNITS IS:
     A. Drug hypersensitivity
     B. Sepsis
     C. Ventilatory failure
     D. Respiratory alkalosis
     E. None of the above
     Ref. Camarata, S. J., Weil, M. H., Hanashiro, P. K., et al: Cardiac
     Arrest in the Critically Ill. I: A Study of Predisposing Causes in 132
     Patients. Circulation, 44:688, 1971.

633. ISOLATION TECHNIQUES AIMED AT EXCLUSION OF AIRBORNE
     TRANSFER OF BACTERIA WOULD BE LEAST EFFECTIVE IN
     PREVENTING INFECTION CAUSED BY:
     A. Streptococci   D. Pneumococci
     B. Hemophilus influenzae   E. C. albicans
     C. P. aeruginosa
     Ref. Ayliffe, G. A. J., Collins, B. J., Lowbury, E. J. L., et al:
     Protective Isolation in Single Bedrooms: Studies in a Modified Hospital
     Ward. J Hyg Camb, 69:511, 1971.

634. WHICH OF THE FOLLOWING ANTIBIOTICS DOES NOT NEUTRALIZE
     GRAM-NEGATIVE ENDOTOXIN?:
     A. Polymyxin B   D. Gentamicin
     B. Polymyxin E   E. Tyrocidine
     C. Colistimethate
     Ref. Corrigan, J. J., Bell, B.: Comparison Between the Polymyxins
     and Gentamicin in Preventing Endotoxin-Induced Intravascular
     Coagulation and Leukopenia. Inf and Imm, 4:563, 1971.

635. THE MOST COMMONLY ENCOUNTERED SIDE EFFECT OF HIGH
     DOSE RIFAMPIN THERAPY (1.2 gm TWICE WEEKLY) IS:
     A. Nausea   D. Thrombocytopenia
     B. Skin rash   E. Fever
     C. Renal failure
     Ref. Poole, G., Stradling, P., Worlledge, S.: Potentially Serious
     Side Effects of High Dose Twice Weekly Rifampin. Brit Med J,
     3:343, 1971.

636.   A DIAGNOSTIC MICROBIOLOGY LABORATORY ROUTINELY USES THE
        DISC DIFFUSION METHOD TO EVALUATE ANTIBIOTIC SENSITIVITY.
        WHICH OF THE FOLLOWING REPORTS SHOULD BE SUSPECTED AS
        BEING INACCURATE?:
        A. N. meningitidis - sensitive to penicillin
        B. B. fragilis - resistant to chloramphenicol
        C. E. coli - sensitive to tetracycline
        D. Enterobacter A - sensitive to cephalothin
        E. P. aeruginosa - resistant to polymyxin B
        Ref. Interpretation of Antimicrobial Susceptibility Tests. The Medical
        Letter, 13:89, 1971.

637.   TETRACYCLINE THERAPY IS ASSOCIATED WITH IMPROVEMENT OF
        WHICH OF THE FOLLOWING TELANGIECTATIC SKIN DISORDERS?:
        A. Rosacea
        B. Scleroderma
        C. Progressive essential telangiectasia
        D. Mastocytosis
        Ref. Shelley, W. B.: Essential Progressive Telangectasia. JAMA,
        216:1343, 1971.

638.   THE PERCENT OF PATIENTS WHO HAVE HAD PRIOR IMMEDIATE
        OR DELAYED HYPERSENSITIVITY RESPONSES TO PENICILLIN AND
        WHO WILL HAVE POSITIVE 30-MINUTE SKIN TEST RESPONSES WHEN
        TESTED WITH PENICILLOYLPOLYLISINE, IS:
        A. 100%   D. 0
        B. 20%   E. 50%
        C. 85%
        Ref. Rosenblum, A. H., Green, G. R.: Cited in Medical News. JAMA,
        215:1906, 1971.

639.   WHAT PERCENT OF AN ORALLY ADMINISTERED 500 mg DOSE OF
        CEPHALEXIN WILL BE EXCRETED IN THE URINE OF NORMAL
        PERSONS WITHIN 6 HOURS OF ADMINISTRATION OF THE ANTIBIOTIC?:
        A. 20   D. 80
        B. 40   E. 90
        C. 60
        Ref. Thornhill, T. S., Levinson, M. E., Johnson, W. D., et al:
        In Vitro Antimicrobial Activity and Human Pharmacology of Cephalexin,
        a New Orally Absorbed Cephalosporin C Antibiotic. Appl Microbiol,
        17:457, 1969.

640.   CARBENICILLIN THERAPY OF PSEUDOMONAS AERUGINOSA
        INFECTIONS HAS BEEN REPORTED TO BE MOST EFFECTIVE WHEN
        THE INFECTION INVOLVES:
        A. Bone
        B. Lung
        C. Bone marrow
        D. Central nervous system
        E. Urinary tract
        Ref. Marks, M. I., Eickhoff, T. C.: Carbenicillin: Clinical and
        Laboratory Evaluation. Ann Intern Med, 73:179, 1970.

641. TWO HOURS AFTER A GROUP OF 3-YEAR-OLDS RECEIVED 12.5 mg OF ERYTHROMYCIN ESTOLATE SUSPENSION, THE MEAN CONCENTRATION IN INFECTED MIDDLE EAR FLUID OBTAINED BY TYMPANOCENTESIS WOULD BE:

A. 0.08 μg
B. 1.30 μg
C. 20 μg
D. 7.5 μg
E. 75 μg

Ref. Bass, J.W., Steele, R.W., Widbe, R.A., et al: Erythromycin Concentrations in Middle Ear Exudates. Pediatrics, 48:417, 1971.

642. WHICH ANTIBIOTIC IS MOST ACTIVE IN VITRO AGAINST AEROMONAS HYDROPHILA?:

A. Gentamicin
B. Ampicillin
C. Cephalothin
D. Carbenicillin
E. Polymyxin B

Ref. Washington, J.A.: Aeromonas Hydrophila in Clinical Bacteriologic Specimens. Ann Intern Med, 76:611, 1972.

643. WHICH OF THE FOLLOWING ANTIBIOTICS IS EFFECTIVE IN TREATING HUMAN INFECTION CAUSED BY GRAM-NEGATIVE ANAEROBIC BACILLI?:

A. Gentamicin
B. Kanamycin
C. Neomycin
D. Framycetin
E. None of the above

Ref. Finegold, S.N., Sutter, V.L.: Susceptibility of Gram-Negative Bacilli to Gentamicin and Other Aminoglycosides. J Inf Dis 124(S):56, 1971.

644. CALCIUM INHIBITS THE EFFECT OF COLISTIN AGAINST WHICH OF THE FOLLOWING ORGANISMS?:

A. P. mirabilis
B. P. vulgaris
C. Klebsiella sp.
D. E. coli
E. P. aeruginosa

Ref. Davis, S.D., Iannetta, A., Wedgwood, R.J.: Activity of Colistin Against Pseudomonas Aeruginosa: Inhibition by Calcium. J Inf Dis, 124:610, 1972.

645. SOME STRAINS OF ENTEROCOCCI ARE RESISTANT TO MORE THAN 5000 μg/ml OF STREPTOMYCIN. WHICH OF THE FOLLOWING ANTIBIOTIC(S) IS MOST LIKELY TO BE INHIBITORY AGAINST THESE HIGHLY RESISTANT STRAINS?:

A. Kanamycin
B. Kanamycin and penicillin
C. Gentamicin and penicillin
D. Ampicillin
E. Vancomycin and ampicillin

Ref. Watanakunakorn, C.: Penicillin Combined with Gentamicin or Streptomycin: Synergism Against Enterococci. J Inf Dis, 124:581, 1971.

646. THE COST OF ANTIMICROBIAL AGENTS USED IN AMERICAN HOSPITALS IN 1972 WILL PROBABLY BE:

A. $815,000,000
B. $246,000,000
C. $103,000,000
D. $400,000,000
E. $100,000,000

Ref. Press, A., Sherman, J.L.: Computerized Review of Antibiotic Therapy. Clinical Medicine, 78:21, 1971.

647.   TREATMENT OF NEONATES WITH GENTAMICIN IS LEAST SATIS-
        FACTORY FOR WHICH OF THE FOLLOWING INFECTIONS?:
        A. Pneumonia   D. Sepsis
        B. Meningitis   E. Pyoderma
        C. Urinary tract infection
        Ref. McCracken, G. H. , Chrane, D. F. , Thomas, M. L. : Pharmacologic
        Evaluation of Gentamicin in Newborn Infants. J Inf Dis, 124(S):214, 1971.

648.   THE DOSE OF GENTAMICIN RECOMMENDED FOR TREATMENT OF
        PSEUDOMONAS BACTEREMIA IN THE INITIAL 24 HOURS, REGARDLESS
        OF RENAL FUNCTIONAL STATE, IS:
        A. .5 mg/kg q 12 h
        B. 6-8 mg/kg in 3 doses
        C. 6-8 mg/kg q 12 h
        D. 2.5 mg/kg in 3 doses
        E. None of the above
        Ref. Jackson, G. G. , Riff, L. J. : Pseudomonas Bacteremia: Pharma-
        cologic and Other Bases for Failure of Treatment with Gentamicin.
        J Inf Dis, 124(S):185, 1971.

649.   IMMEDIATELY FOLLOWING INTRAVENOUS ADMINISTRATION OF
        AMPHOTERICIN B:
        A. 60% of the administered dose is present in the serum
        B. Concentration in tissues parallels concentration in serum
        C. 90% of the drug appears in the urine in a biologically active form
        D. Most of the drug is inactivated or stored
        Ref. Bindschadler, D. D. , Bennett, J. E. : A Pharmacologic Guide to the
        Clinical Use of Amphotericin B. J Infect Dis, 120:427, 1969.

650.   WHICH OF THE FOLLOWING ANTIBIOTICS IS MOST ACTIVE AGAINST
        KLEBSIELLA PNEUMONIAE?:
        A. Tetracycline   D. Streptomycin
        B. Gentamicin   E. Cephalothin
        C. Ampicillin
        Ref. Martin, W. J. , Yu, P. K. W. , Washington, J. A. : Epidemiologic
        Significance of Klebsiella Pneumoniae: A 3 Month Study. Mayo Clin
        Proc, 46:785, 1971.

651.   WHICH OF THE FOLLOWING ASPECTS OF FRACTURE HEALING
        IS DISTURBED BY OXYTETRACYCLINE ADMINISTRATION?:
        A. Tensile strength of callus
        B. Mineral concentration of callus
        C. 24 hour uptake of radioactive strontium by callus
        D. Breaking strength of fracture callus
        E. Total collagen concentration
        Ref. Gudmundson, C. : Oxytetracycline-Induced Disturbance of
        Fracture Healing. J Trauma, 11:511, 1971.

652.   AFTER DAILY INJECTIONS OF 2.5 mg OF POLYMYXIN B/kg BODY
        WEIGHT IN THE RABBIT, WHICH OF THE FOLLOWING STATEMENTS
        IS MORE NEARLY CORRECT?:
        A. Gradual accumulation of free polymyxin B in serum
        B. Gradual accumulation of free polymyxin B in the lung
        C. Muscle will accumulate the highest concentrations of bound polymyxin B
        D. The kidney will accumulate more bound polymyxin B than the muscle
        E. Essentially no bound polymyxin B will be recovered from muscle or
            kidney 48 hours after the last dose of polymyxin B
        Ref. Kunin, C. M. , Bugg, A. : Binding of Polymyxin Antibiotics to
        Tissues: The Major Determinant of Distribution and Persistance in the
        Body. J Infect Dis, 124:394, 1971.

653.   THE GEOMETRIC MEAN CONCENTRATION (μg/ml) OF GENTAMICIN
        NECESSARY TO INHIBIT 90% OF PSEUDOMONAS AERUGINOSA
        STRAINS ISOLATED FROM INFECTED HUMANS IS:
        A. 0.5   D. 12.5
        B. 1   E. 25 or greater
        C. 3.2
        Ref. Young, L. S.: Gentamicin: Clinical Use with Carbenicillin and
        In Vitro Studies with Recent Isolates of Pseudomonas Aeruginosa.
        J Inf Dis, 124(S):202, 1971.

654.   ORAL AMPHOTERICIN B HAS BEEN USED SUCCESSFULLY IN THE
        TREATMENT OF:
        A. Chronic mucocutaneous candidiasis
        B. Musculoskeletal coccidioidomycosis
        C. Facial blastomycosis
        D. Cryptococcosis
        E. All of the above
        Ref. Montes, L. F., Cooper, M. D., Bradford, R. O., et al: Prolonged
        Oral Treatment of Chronic Mucocutaneous Candidiasis with Amphotericin
        B. Arch Derm, 104:45, 1971.

655.   THE MOST IMPORTANT MECHANISM OF RESISTANCE TO GENTAMICIN
        AMONG PSEUDOMONAS AERUGINOSA STRAINS ISOLATED UNDER
        NATURAL CONDITIONS IS:
        A. Alteration of ribosomes
        B. Gentamicin inactiviting enzymes
        C. Altered permeability to gentamicin
        D. Inactivation due to R factors
        E. None of the above
        Ref. Davies, J.: Bacterial Resistance to Aminoglycoside Antibiotics.
        J Inf Dis, 124(S):7, 1971.

656.   ONE HOUR AFTER INGESTING 250 mg (400,000 UNITS) OF POTASSIUM
        PENICILLIN-V IN THE FASTING STATE, THE SERUM LEVEL
        (MICROGRAMS/ml) OF PENICILLIN WOULD BE EXPECTED TO BE:
        A. .03   D. 1.8
        B. 30   E. 18
        C. .15
        Ref. Fishman, L. S., Hewitt, W. L.: The Natural Penicillins.
        Med Clin N Amer, 54:1081, 1970.

657.   FOR HOW MANY WEEKS IS PENICILLIN DETECTABLE IN THE SERUM
        AFTER A SINGLE INTRAMUSCULAR INJECTION OF 1.2 MILLION UNITS
        OF BENZATHINE PENICILLIN?:
        A. 1   D. 4
        B. 2   E. 6
        C. 3
        Ref. Fishman, L. S., Hewitt, W. L.: The Natural Penicillins.
        Med Clin N Amer, 54:1081, 1970.

658.   THE COST TO THE PATIENT OF 10 DAYS THERAPY AT RECOMMENDED
        DOSES WOULD BE HIGHEST WITH WHICH OF THE FOLLOWING
        ANTIBIOTICS?:
        A. Sulfisoxazole   D. Triple sulfas
        B. Doxycycline   E. Cephalexin
        C. Tetracycline
        Ref. Hand Book of Antimicrobial Therapy. The Medical Letter,
        14:51, 1972.

659. IT HAS BEEN SUGGESTED THAT PATIENTS WITH INFECTIOUS
      MONONUCLEOSIS OR LYMPHATIC LEUKEMIA SHOULD NOT RECEIVE
      AMPICILLIN UNLESS IT IS CLEARLY NECESSARY BECAUSE OF:
      A. Hypogammaglobulinemia
      B. Hypersensitivity reactions
      C. Staphylococcal suprainfections
      D. Ampicillin is not effective against P. aeruginosa
      E. None of the above
      Ref. Cameron, S.J., Richmond, J.: Ampicillin Hypersensitivity in
      Lymphatic Leukemia. Scot Med J, 16:425, 1971.

660. THE ANTIBIOTIC(S) PRODUCING THE MOST EFFECTIVE ANTI-
      BACTERIAL ACTIVITY IN EXPERIMENTAL PYELONEPHRITIS OF
      THE RAT CAUSED BY GROUP D STREPTOCOCCI IS (ARE):
      A. Penicillin
      B. Penicillin and streptomycin
      C. Streptomycin
      D. Ampicillin
      E. Ampicillin and streptomycin
      Ref. Sapico, F.L., Kalmanson, G.M., Montgomerie, J.Z., et al:
      Pyelonephritis XII. Comparison of Penicillin, Ampicillin and
      Streptomycin in Enterococcal Infection in Rats. J Infec Dis,
      123:611, 1971.

661. THE MOST COMMON ORGANISM COLONIZING BURNED PATIENTS
      TREATED WITH GENTAMICIN IS:
      A. C. albicans
      B. Gentamicin-resistant P. aeruginosa
      C. S. aureus
      D. Serratia sp.
      E. E. coli
      Ref. MacMillan, B.G.: Ecology of Bacteria Colonizing the Burned
      Patient Given Topical and Systemic Gentamicin Therapy: A Five Year
      Study. J Inf Dis, 124(S):278, 1971.

662. ANTIBIOTIC ASSAY SYSTEMS RECENTLY DEVELOPED MAY ALLOW
      ESTIMATION OF CONCENTRATIONS OF GENTAMICIN, KANAMYCIN
      OR STREPTOMYCIN IN THE SERUM AS SOON AS:
      A. 20 minutes   D. 24 hours
      B. 4 hours   E. None of the above
      C. 12 hours
      Ref. Sabath, L.D., Casey, J.I., Ruch, P.A., Stumpf, L.L.,
      Finland, M.: Rapid Microassay of Gentamicin, Kanamycin, Neomycin,
      Streptomycin, and Vancomycin in Serum or Plasma. J Lab Clin Med,
      78:457, 1971.

663. WHICH OF THE FOLLOWING ANTIBIOTICS IS USUALLY AVOIDED
      EVEN AT REDUCED DOSE FOR THE TREATMENT OF INFECTION IN
      THE UREMIC PATIENT?:
      A. Ampicillin   D. Carbenicillin
      B. Lincomycin   E. Tetracycline
      C. Erythromycin
      Ref. Bulger, R.J., Petersdorf, R.G.: Antimicrobial Therapy in
      Patients with Renal Insufficiency. Postgrad Med J, 47:160, 1970.

664. WHICH OF THE FOLLOWING ARE CAUSED BY TETRACYCLINE
      THERAPY?:
      A. Photophobia
      B. Pruritis
      C. Gastrointestinal disturbances
      D. Benign intracranial hypertension
      E. All of the above
      Ref. Maroon, J. C. , Mealy, J. , Jr. : Benign Intracranial Hypertension.
      JAMA, 216:1479, 1971.

665. WHICH OF THE FOLLOWING ANTIBIOTICS ATTAINS THE HIGHEST
      CONCENTRATION IN CEREBROSPINAL FLUID WHERE BACTERIAL
      MENINGITIS IS PRESENT?:
      A. Methicillin
      B. Cephalothin
      C. Cephaloridine
      Ref. Oppenheimer, S. , Beaty, H. N. , Petersdorf, R. G. : Pathogenesis
      of Meningitis VIII. Cerebrospinal Fluid and Blood Concentrations of
      Methicillin, Cephalothin and Cephaloridine in Experimental
      Pneumococcal Meningitis. J Lab Clin Med, 73:535, 1969.

666. THE GENTAMICIN HALF-LIFE IN HOURS CAN BE ESTIMATED BY
      MULTIPLYING THE SERUM CREATININE BY:
      A. .25   D. 0.1
      B. 9   E. 8
      C. 4
      Ref. Cutler, R. E. , Gyselynck, A. M. , Fleet, W. P. , et al: Correlation
      of Serum Creatinine Concentration and Gentamicin Half-Life. JAMA,
      219:1037, 1972.

667. WHICH OF THE FOLLOWING SEMI-SYNTHETIC PENICILLINS IS
      LEAST BOUND TO SERUM ALBUMIN?:
      A. Dicloxacillin   D. Methicillin
      B. Cloxacillin   E. Nafcillin
      C. Oxacillin
      Ref. Gilbert, D. N. , Sanford, J. P. : Methicillin: Critical Appraisal
      After a Decade of Experience. Med Clin N Amer, 54:1113, 1970.

668. TWO HOURS AFTER A SINGLE INTRAVENOUS DOSE OF METHICILLIN,
      THE SERUM CONCENTRATION IN A PATIENT WITH NORMAL RENAL
      AND HEPATIC FUNCTION WOULD BE APPROXIMATELY (IN
      MICROGRAMS/ml):
      A. 70   D. 10
      B. 5   E. None of the above
      C. .05
      Ref. Gilbert, D. N. , Sanford, J. P. : Methicillin: Critical Appraisal
      After a Decade of Experience. Med Clin N Amer, 54:1113, 1970.

669. THE MAJORITY OF STRAINS OF THE FOLLOWING GRAM-NEGATIVE
      BACTERIA WOULD BE EXPECTED TO BE SUSCEPTIBLE TO POLYMYXIN
      B SULFATE (10 MICROGRAMS/ml), EXCEPT:
      A. Klebsiella sp.   D. Hemophilus sp.
      B. Proteus sp.   E. Pseudomonas sp.
      C. Escherichia sp.
      Ref. Goodwin, N. J. , Colistin and Sodium Colistimethate. Med Clin
      N Amer, 54:1267, 1970.

670. AMPICILLIN IS THE DRUG OF CHOICE FOR TREATMENT OF ADULTS
WITH:
 A. Bacterial sepsis of unknown etiology
 B. Chronic bacteruria
 C. Purulent exacerbations of chronic bronchitis
 D. Bacteroides sp. infections
 E. None of the above
Ref. Bear, D. M. , Turck, M. , Petersdorf, R. G.: Ampicillin.
Med Clin N Amer, 54:1145, 1970.

671. THE MOST COMMONLY PRESCRIBED CLASSES OF DRUGS IN A
COMMUNITY NON-UNIVERSITY HOSPITAL SETTING ARE:
 A. Amphetamines
 B. Tranquilizers
 C. Antibiotics
 D. Non-narcotic analgesics
 E. Contraceptive steroids
Ref. Stolley, P. D. , Becker, M. H. , McEvilla, J. D. , et al: Drug
Prescribing and Use in an American Community. Ann Intern Med,
76:537, 1972.

THE FOLLOWING QUESTIONS CONSIST OF PAIRS OF PHRASES
DESCRIBING CONDITIONS OR QUANTITIES WHICH MAY OR MAY NOT
VARY IN RELATION TO EACH OTHER. ANSWER:
 A. If increase in the first is accompanied by increase in the second or
   decrease in the first is accompanied by decrease in the second
 B. If increase in the first is accompanied by decrease in the second or
   decrease in the first is accompanied by increase in the second
 C. If changes in the first are independent of changes in the second

672. 1. Number of bacterial infections in Chediak-Higashi syndrome
  2. Number of prophylactic courses of cloxacillin
Ref. Dale, D. C. , Alling, D. W. , Wolff, S. M.: Cloxacillin Chemoprophylaxis in the Chediak-Higashi syndrome. J Inf Dis, 125:393, 1972.

673. 1. Total number of children with lobar pneumonia who will respond
    favorably to antibiotic therapy within 48 hours of treatment
  2. Total leukocyte count
Ref. Shuttleworth, D. B. , Charney, E.: Leukocyte Count in Childhood
Pneumonia. Amer J Dis Child, 122:393, 1971.

674. 1. Serum half-life of kanamycin
  2. Serum creatinine
Ref. McCloskey, R. V. , Becker, G. G.: Evaluation of the Cutler-Orme
Method for the Administration of Kanamycin During Renal Failure.
Antimicrob Agents Chemotherap, 1970, pp. 161-164, American Society for
Microbiology, 1971.

675. 1. Frequency of hemodialysis
  2. Serum $T\frac{1}{2}$ of doxycycline
Ref. Mannhart, M. , Dettli, L. , Spring, P.: Doxycycline Elimination and
its Modification by Hemodialysis in Anuric Patients. Schweiz Med Wschr,
101:123, 1971.

676. 1. Sensitivity of tobramycin assay
  2. Percent sodium in agar used to assay tobramycin
Ref. Lamb, J. W. , Mann, J. M. , Simmon, R. J.: Factors Influencing the
Microbiological Assay of Tobramycin. Antimicro Ag Chem, 1:323, 1972.

677.   1.   Number of patients treated with carbenicillin in a given hospital
       2.   Numbers of isolates of P. aeruginosa in that hospital which produce
            a beta lactamase
       Ref. Ayliffe, G. A. J., Lowbury, E. J. L., Roe, E.: Transferable
       Carbenicillin Resistance in Pseudomonas Aeruginosa. Nature, 235:141,
       1972.

678.   1.   Treatment of a given population with rifampin for gonorrhea
       2.   Number of gonococcal strains resistant to rifampin isolated from
            that population
       Ref. Malmborg, A-S, Molin, L., Nystrom, B.: Rifampicin Compared
       with Penicillin in the Treatment of Gonorrhea. Chemother, 16:319, 1971.

679.   1.   Resistance of P. aeruginosa to gentamicin
       2.   Resistance of P. aeruginosa to tobramycin
       Ref. Brusdi, J. L., Barza, M., Bergeron, M. G., et al: Cross-
       Resistance of Pseudomonas to Gentamicin and Tobramycin.
       Antimicrob Ag Chemother, 1:280, 1972.

680.   1.   MBC of cephapirin
       2.   Number of bacteria in inoculum
       Ref. Wiesner, P., MacGregor, R., Bear, D., et al: Evaluation of a
       New Cephalosporin Antibiotic, Cephapirin. Antimicrob Ag Chemother,
       1:303, 1972.

681.   1.   Elimination constant for gentamicin
       2.   Sustaining dose of gentamicin needed to produce inhibitory non-toxic
            serum concentrations
       Ref. Chan, R. A., Benner, E. J., Hoeprich, P. D.: Gentamicin Therapy
       in Renal Failure: A Nomogram for Dosage. Ann Intern Med, 76:773, 1972.

682.   1.   Serum half-time of carbencillin
       2.   Creatinine clearance
       Ref. Hoffmann, T. A., Cestero, R., Bullock, W. E.: Pharmacodynamics
       of Carbenicillin in Hepatic and Renal Failure. Ann Intern Med, 73:173,
       1970.

683.   1.   Inflammation of the meninges
       2.   Penetration of cephaloridine into the CSF
       Ref. Lerner, P. I.: Penetration of Cephaloridine Into Cerebrospinal
       Fluid. Amer J Med Sci, 262:321, 1972.

684.   1.   Use of antibacterial ointments or pads at site of entry of intravenous
            polyethylene catheters
       2.   Percent of catheter tip cultures which contain bacteria
       Ref. Crenshaw, C. A., Kelly, L. A., Turner, R. J., III: Bacteriologic
       Nature and Prevention of Contamination to Intravenous Catheters.
       Amer J Surg, 123:264, 1972.

685.   1. pH of urine
       2. Ampicillin crystalluria
       Ref. Potter, J. L., Weinberg, A. G., West, R.: Ampicillinuria and
       Ampicillin Crystaluria. Pediatrics, 48:636, 1971.

686.   1. Hematocrit
        2. Gentamicin serum concentration
        Ref. Riff, L. J., Jackson, G. G.: Pharmacology of Gentamicin in Man.
        J Inf Dis, 124(S):98, 1971.

687.   1. Serum half-time of carbenicillin
        2. Hepatic dysfunction
        Ref. Hoffman, T. A., Cestero, R., Bullock, W. E.: Pharmacodynamics
        of Carbenicillin in Hepatic and Renal Failure. Ann Intern Med, 73:173,
        1970.

688.   1. Renal function
        2. Serum level of doxycycline using conventional dose schedules
        Ref. Morgan, T., Ribush, N.: Effect of Oxytetracycline and Doxycycline
        on Protein Metabolism. Med J Aust, 1:55, 1972.

THE FOLLOWING QUESTIONS CONSIST OF A STATEMENT AND A
REASON. SELECT:
A. If both statement and reason are true and the reason is a correct
    explanation of the statement
B. If both statement and reason are true but the reason is not a correct
    explanation of the statement
C. If the statement is true but the reason is false
D. If the statement is false but the reason is true
E. If both statement and reason are false

689. ___ Steroids do not contribute to survival from Gram negative bacillary
        sepsis BECAUSE double blind studies show that the survival of septic
        patients receiving betamethasone is no greater than septic patients
        receiving placebo medication.
        Ref. Plotkin, S. A.: Antibiotics, 1971. Clin Ped, 10:369, 1971.

690. ___ Antimicrobial therapy is indicated for treatment of all streptococcal
        pharyngitis and pyoderma BECAUSE antimicrobial therapy has been
        shown to reduce the risk of glomerulonephritis following streptococcosis.
        Ref. Weinstein, L., LeFrock, J.: Does Antimicrobial Therapy of
        Streptococcal Pharyngitis or Pyoderma Alter the Risk of Glomerulone-
        phritis. J Inf Dis, 124:229, 1971.

691. ___ Some authorities consider tetracyclines to be the drugs of choice for
        the treatment of gonorrhea BECAUSE penicillin given for gonorrhea
        may abort incubating syphilis.
        Ref. Neumann, H. H., Baecker, J. M.: Treatment of Gonorrhea.
        JAMA, 219:471, 1972.

692. ___ Pentamidine isethionate is recommended for treatment of pneumonia-
        caused Pneumocystis carinii BECAUSE pentamidine isethionate is the
        only known agent effective against Pneumocystis carinii.
        Ref. Kirby, H. B., Kenamore, B., Guckian, J. C.: Pneumocystis
        Carini Pneumonia Treated with Pyrimethamine and Sulfadiazine.
        Ann Intern Med, 75:505-509, 1971.

693. ___ Freshly prepared benzyl penicillin G is unsatisfactory as an antigen for skin testing to evaluate penicillin hypersensitivity BECAUSE false positive skin reactions to freshly prepared benzyl penicillin G are common.
Ref. Fishman, L. S., Hewitt, W. L.: The Natural Penicillins.
Med Clin N Amer, 54:1081, 1970.

694. ___ Long-acting sulfonamides such as sulfadimethoxine or sulfamethoxypy-ridazine are usually not recommended for urinary tract infection therapy BECAUSE the long-acting sulfonamides are accompanied by a higher incidence of toxic reactions than are trisulfapyrimidines or sulfisoxazole.
Ref. Pryles, C. V.: The Use of Sulfonamides in Urinary Tract Infection.
Med Clin N Amer, 54:1077, 1970.

695. ___ Most authorities recommend penicillin for prophylaxis of meningococcal infection BECAUSE many strains of meningococci are now resistant to sulfonamides.
Ref. Handbook of Antimicrobial Therapy. The Medical Letter, 14:30, 1972.

696. Gentamicin is a valuable drug for the treatment of neonatal sepsis BECAUSE urinary excretion of the drug is rapid in the first week of life.
Ref. Plotkin, S. A.: Antibiotics, 1971. Clin Ped, 10:369, 1971.

697. ___ Gentamicin has an excellent spectrum of activity against Gram negative bacilli BECAUSE the blood level that can safely be achieved is not much higher than the therapeutic level.
Ref. Plotkin, S. A.: Antibiotics, 1971. Clin Ped, 10:369, 1971.

698. ___ The initial dose of cephalexin for treatment of infection in a patient with severe renal insufficiency should be that precribed for a normal subject BECAUSE if the first dose of cephalexin is reduced in renal insufficiency, there will be a delay in achieving effective serum concentrations.
Ref. Regamez, C., Humair, L.: Pharmokinetics of Cephalexin in Renal Insufficiency. Postgrad Med J, Feb Supp: 69, 1971.

699. ___ Minocycline and rifampin administration both reduce meningococcal carrier rates BECAUSE rifampin-resistant organisms are encountered after rifampin therapy for the meningococcal carrier state.
Ref. Guttler, R., Counts, G. W., Avent, C. K., Beaty, H. N.: Effect of Rifampin and Minocycline on Meningococcal Carrier Rates.
J Infec Dis, 124:199, 1971.

700. ___ The use of carbenicillin (400 mg/kg/day) and gentamicin (5 mg/kg/day) does not eliminate P. aeruginosa from the sputum of patients with cystic fibrosis BECAUSE the MIC for these organisms is higher than the concentration of either antibiotic attained in the sputum.
Ref. Marks, M. I., Prentice, R., Swarson, R., et al: Carbenicillin and Gentamicin: Pharmacologic Studies in Patients with Cystic Fibrosis and Pseudomonas Pulmonary Infections. J Ped, 79:822, 1971.

701. ___ The recommended initial dose of gentamicin for bacteremic life-threatening infection is 7-8 mg/kg BECAUSE the hematocrit is related to the concentration of gentamicin attained in the serum.
Ref. Riff, L. J., Jackson, G. G.: Pharmacology of Gentamicin in Man. J Inf Dis, 124(S):98, 1971.

702. ___ Patients treated for gonorrhea with spectinomycin or tetracycline should have serologic tests for syphilis monthly for 4 months BECAUSE spectinomycin and tetracycline are not considered as adequate therapy for incubating syphilis.
Ref. Morbidity and Mortality, 21:82, 1972.

703. ___ Tetracycline (3 gm daily) has no beneficial effect on the ocular signs of trachoma BECAUSE this regimen has no effect on the incidence of chalmydia present in conjunctival scrapings.
Ref. Dawson, C. R., Ostler, H. B., Hanna, L., et al: Tetracycline in the Treatment of Chronic Trachoma in American Indians. J Inf Dis, 124:255, 1971.

704. ___ Carbenicillin is effective in the treatment of Pseudomonas aeruginosa BECAUSE most strains of Pseudomonas aeruginosa are highly sensitive to this antibiotic in vitro.
Ref. Solberg, C. O., Kjellstrand, K. M., Matsen, J. N.: Carbenicillin Therapy of Severe Pseudomonas Aeruginosa Infections. J Chron Dis, 24:19, 1971.

705. ___ It is desirable that all laboratories adopt a uniform method for testing antibiotic sensitivity BECAUSE variations in drug content of discs and inoculum size may lead to an organism being identified as sensitive by one hospital and resistant by another.
Ref. Castle, A. R., Elstub, J.: Antibiotic Sensitivity Testing: A Survey Undertaken in September 1970 in the United Kingdom. J Clin Path, 24:773, 1971.

706. ___ Systemic antibiotic therapy should not be used in an attempt to prevent infection of indwelling venous cannulae BECAUSE neither local or systemic antibiotic therapy reduce the risk of septic thrombophlebitis.
Ref. McHaffie, D. J.: Sepsis and Intravenous Catheters. New Zealand Med J, 74:164, 1971.

707. ___ Ampicillin - sulfonamide therapy is successful in the treatment of pulmonary nocardiosis BECAUSE synergism can be demonstrated by testing nocardia species against ampicillin and sulfonamides in vitro.
Ref. Orfanakis, M. G., Wilcox, H. G., Smith, C. B.: In Vitro Studies of the Combined Effect of Ampicillin and Sulfonamides on Nocardia Asteroides and Results of Therapy in Four Patients. Antimicrob Ag Chemother, 1:215, 1972.

708. ___ In most instances, orally administered lincomycin should not be used to treat infected patients with severe liver disease BECAUSE orally administered lincomycin is excreted primarily into the bile.
Ref. Sanders, E.: Lincomycin: Fact, Fancy and Future. Med Clin N Amer, 54:1295, 1970.

709. ___ Coombs-positive hemolytic anemia is commonly seen during cephalothin therapy BECAUSE over 50% of patients receiving cephalothin develop a positive direct Coombs' test.
Ref. Gralnick, H. R., McGinniss, M., Elton, W., et al: Hemolytic Anemia Associated with Cephalothin. JAMA, 217:1193, 1971.

710. ___ An organism reported as resistant to colistin sulfate would be expected to be sensitive to polymyxin B sulfate BECAUSE cross resistance of organisms to polymyxin B sulfate and colistin sulfate is uncommon.
Ref. Goodwin, N. J.: Colistin and Sodium Colistimethate. Med Clin N Amer, 54:1271, 1970.

711. ___ Rifampin is effective in the elimination of meningococci from the nasopharynx BECAUSE the minimum inhibitory concentration for most meningococcal strains is less than the concentration of rifampin in saliva 3-4 hours after a third 600 mg dose of rifampin.
Ref. Devine, L. F., Johnson, D. P., Hagerman, C. R., et al, Rafampin. JAMA, 214:1055, 1970.

712. ___ Gonorrhea patients treated with the usually recommended short course of tetracycline should have 3 monthly serologic tests for syphilis BECAUSE this tetracycline regimen will not abort all cases of incubating syphilis.
Ref. Lucas, J. B.: Gonococcal Resistance to Antibiotics. South Med Bull, 59:22, 1971.

713. ___ Patients with gonorrhea who have received 2.4 or 4.8 million units of aqueous procaine penicillin G do not require monthly serologic tests for syphilis BECAUSE those doses of penicillin will also cure any coexisting incubating syphilis.
Ref. Lucas, J. B.: Gonococcal Resistance to Antiobiotics. South Med Bull, 59:22, 1971.

714. ___ Trimethroprin and sulfamethoxazole, used jointly, are effective in treating gonorrhea in women BECAUSE most strains of N. gonorrhoeae are not resistant to sulfonamides.
Ref. Schofield. C. B. S., Masterton, G., Moffett, M., et al: Gonorrhea in Women: Treatment with Sulfamethoxazole and Trimethoprin. J Inf Dis, 124:533, 1971.

715. ___ Patients with chronic bronchitis do not harbor the same pneumococcal type in the sputum for more than a few weeks BECAUSE pneumococci are easily eliminated from the sputum of chronic bronchitis using antibiotic therapy.
Ref. Calder, M. E., Schonell, M. E.: Pneumococcal Typing and the Problem of Endogenous or Exogenous Reinfection in Chronic Bronchitis. Lancet, 1:1156, 1971.

716. ___ Chloramphenicol is the drug of choice for treatment of typhoid fever BECAUSE less than 10% of S. typhi strains tested are sensitive to a combination of trimethoprim and sulfamethoxazole.
Ref. Scragg, J. N., Rubidge, C. J.: Trimethoprim and Sulfamethoxazole in Typhoid Fever in Children. Brit Med J, 3:738, 1971.

717. ___ In experimental staphylococcal osteomyelitis in rabbits, cephalothin is less effective when given for 4 weeks than lincomycin BECAUSE cephalothin levels in diseased bone are lower than lincomycin levels.
Ref. Norden, C. W.: Experimental Osteomyelitis II Therapeutic Trials and Measurement of Antibiotic Levels in Bone. J Inf Dis, 124:565, 1971.

718. ___ An otherwise healthy adult with symptomatic salmonella enteritis should be treated with trimethoprim and sulfamethoxazole BECAUSE this treatment will shorten the duration of symptoms and reduce their severity.
Ref. Smith, E. R., Badley, B. W. D.: Treatment of Salmonella Enteritis and its Effect on Carrier State. Canad Med Assoc J, 104:1004, 1971.

719. ___ The routine use of antibiotics prior to and during closed heart surgery is not justified BECAUSE the incidence of infection is higher in those receiving antibiotics.
Sallam, I. A., et al: Prophylactic Antibiotics and Closed Heart Surgery. Chest, 60:252, 1971.

720. ___ In vitro testing of Pseudomonas sp. sensitivity to polymyxins and carbenicillin is a useful guide to therapy BECAUSE in vitro sensitivity testing is directly related to the therapeutic response.
Ref. Bodey, G. P., Whitecar, J. P., Middleman, E., et al: Carbenicillin Therapy for Pseudomonas Infections. JAMA, 218:62, 1971.

721. ___ The strains of E. coli responsible for uncomplicated acute urinary tract infections are usually sensitive to a wide variety of antibiotics effective against Gram-negative organisms BECAUSE the E. coli causing the infection is very often serologically related to strains of E. coli in the patients' stool.
Ref. Wallace, J. F., Petersdorf, R. G.: Urinary Tract Infections. Postgrad Med, 50:138, 1971.

722. ___ Rifampin is an effective antibiotic for the elimination of the meningococcal carrier state BECAUSE the concentration of rifampin in the saliva approaches the in vitro minimal inhibiting concentration of the meningococcus.
Ref. Devine, L. F., Rhode, S. L., Pierce, W. E., et al: Rifampin: Effect of a Two Day Treatment Plan on the Meningococcal Carrier State and the Relationship to the Levels of the Drug in Sera and Saliva. Amer J Med Sci, 261:79, 1971.

723. ___ Penicillin is the drug of choice for the treatment of pneumococcal pneumonia BECAUSE pneumococci partially resistant to penicillin have never been isolated from humans.
Ref. Hansman, D., Glasgow, H., Sturt, J., et al: Increased Resistance to Penicillin of Pneumococci Isolated from Man. New Eng J Med, 284:175, 1971.

724. ___ Intraarticular administration of Ampicillin, methicillin, or penicillin is required in treating septic arthritides caused by bacteria sensitive to these antibiotics BECAUSE Ampicillin, methicillin, and penicillin administered by parenteral routes do not attain concentrations inhibitory to bacteria usually responsible for septic arthritis.
Ref. Nelson, J. D.: Antibiotic Concentrations in Septic Joint Effusions. New Eng J Med, 284:349, 1971.

725. ___ There is general agreement that as clinical improvement occurs during the course of H. influenzae meningitis, the dose of ampicillin should not be reduced BECAUSE penetration of ampicillin into the CSF declines as meningeal irritation abates.
Ref. Haltalin, K. C. , Smith, J. B. : Reevaluation of Ampicillin Therapy for Hemophilus Influenzae Meningitis. Am J Dis Child, 122:328, 1971.

726. ___ Iodochlorhydroxyquin (Entero-vioform) does not prevent travelers' diarrhea BECAUSE the specific cause of travelers' diarrhea is enteropathogenic E. coli.
Ref. Schultz, M. G. : Entero-Vioform for Preventing Travelers' Diarrhea. JAMA, 220:273, 1972.

ANSWER THE FOLLOWING QUESTIONS ACCORDING TO THE KEY BELOW:
A. If choice A is greater than choice B
B. If choice B is greater than choice A
C. If A and B are equal or nearly equal

727. MICROBIOLOGIC ACTIVITY OF GENTAMICIN IN:
A. Unheparinized blood
B. Therapeutically heparinized blood
Ref. Regamey, C. , Schaberg, D. , Kirby, W. M. M. : Inhibitory Effect of Heparin on Gentamicin Concentrations in Blood. Antimicrob Ag Chemother, 1:329, 1972.

728. SERUM CONCENTRATION OF (mcg/ml) OF:
A. Amoxicillin 2 hours after oral ingestion of 500 mg of amoxicillin
B. Ampicillin 2 hours after oral ingestion of 500 mg of ampicillin
Ref. Bodey, G. P. , Nance, J. : Amoxicillin: In Vitro and Pharmacologic Studies. Antimicrob Ag Chemother, 1:358, 1972.

729. CARBENICILLIN $T_{\frac{1}{2}}$ IN SERUM
A. Between hemodialysis
B. During dialysis
Ref. Kirby, W. M. M. : Antimicrobial Management of Gram-Negative Sepsis in Gram-Negative Sepsis. Sanford, J. P. , (ed), Med Com, New York, N. Y. , 1972, p. 64.

730. FAILURE RATE IN TREATING GONORRHEA OF MEN OR WOMEN WITH A SINGLE DOSE OF:
A. 900 mgm of rifampin
B. 2.5 megaunits of penicillin
Ref. Malmborg, A-S, Molin, L. , Nystrom, B. , Rifampicin Compared with Penicillin in the Treatment of Gonorrhea. Chemother, 16:319, 1971.

731. SERUM $T_{\frac{1}{2}}$ OF CARBENICILLIN IN PATIENTS WITH:
A. Renal failure
B. Renal failure with hepatic dysfunction
Ref. Hoffman, T. A. , Cestero, R. , Bullock, W. E. : Pharmacodynamics of Carbenicillin in Hepatic and Renal Failure. Ann Intern Med, 73:173, 1970.

732. RATIO OF CSF TO SERUM CONCENTRATION DURING ADMINIS-TRATION OF:
A. Amphotericin B
B. Flucytosine
Ref. The Medical Letter, 14:29, 1972.

733.   ACTIVITY AGAINST PSEUDOMONAS OF:
        A. Carbenicillin indanyl sodium
        B. Carbenicillin disodium
        Ref. English, A. R. , Retsma, J. A. , Ray, V. A. : Carbenicillin Indanyl
        Sodium, an Orally Active Derivative of Carbenicillin. Antimicrob Ag
        Chemother, 1:185, 1972.

734.   THE ANTIBACTERIAL SPECTRUM OF:
        A. Cephapirin
        B. Cephalothin
        Ref. Axelrod, J. , Meyers, B. R. , Hirshman, S. Z. : Cephapirin:
        Pharmacology in Normal Volunteers, J Clin Pharm, 12:84, 1972.

735.   STABILITY OF AMPICILLIN IN INTRAVENOUS SOLUTION OF:
        A. pH 8.5
        B. pH 6.9
        Ref. Wyatt, R. G. , Okamato, G. A. , Feigin, R. D. : Stability of
        Antibiotics in Parenteral Solutions. Pediatrics, 49:22, 1972.

736.   RELAPSE RATE OF WOMEN TREATED FOR GONORRHEA WITH:
        A. 4.8 megaunits of procaine penicillin G
        B. 4 gm of spectinomycin
        Ref. Pedersen, A. H. , Weisner, P. J. , Holmes, K. H. , et al:
        Spectinomycin and Penicillin G in the Treatment of Gonorrhea. JAMA,
        220:205, 1972.

737.   EFFECTIVENESS OF THE FOLLOWING DRUGS IN TREATING SHIGEL-
        LOSIS AFFECTING CHILDREN:
        A. Furazolidone
        B. Ampicillin
        Ref. Haltalin, K. C. , Nelson, J. D. : Failure of Furazolidone Therapy
        in Shigellosis. Am J Dis Child, 123:40, 1972.

738.   RECOVERY RATE OF CHILDREN WITH PERTUSSIS TREATED WITH:
        A. Ampicillin
        B. Ampicillin plus pertussis immune globulin
        Ref. Balagtos, R. C. : Treatment of Pertussis with Pertussis Immune
        Globulin. J Pediatr, 79:203, 1971.

739.   SERUM T$\frac{1}{2}$ OF CEPHAPIRIN IN:UREMIC PATIENTS:
        A. Receiving extracorporeal dialysis
        B. Not being dialyzed
        Ref. McCloskey, R. V. , Terry, E. E. , McCracken, A. , et al: Effect of
        Hemodialysis and Renal Failure on Serum and Urine Concentrations of
        Cephapirin Sodium. Antimicrob Ag Chemother, 1:90, 1972.

740.   ZONE OF INHIBITION AROUND AN AMPICILLIN SENSITIVE ORGANISM
        USING STANDARD AMPICILLIN DISCS FOR SENSITIVITY TESTING ON:
        A. Trypticase Soy Agar
        B. Trypticase Soy Agar - 5% sheep blood (defibrinated)
        Ref. Brenner, V. C. , Sherris, J. C. : Influence of Different Media and
        Bloods on the Results of Diffusion Antibiotic Susceptibility Tests.
        Antimicrob Ag Chemother, 1:116, 1972.

741.   MIC OF ERYTHROMYCIN AND LINCOMYCIN AGAINST BACTEROIDES
        FRAGILIS:
        A. In hydrogen atmosphere
        B. In hydrogen - CO_2 atmosphere
        Ref. Ingham, H. R. , Selkon, J. B. , Codd, A. A. , et al: The Effect of
        Carbon dioxide on the Sensitivity of Bacteroides Fragilis to Certain
        Antibiotics in Vitro. J Clin Path, 23:254, 1970.

742. REMOVAL BY DIALYSIS OF
A. Polymyxin B, sulfate
B. Polymyxin E, sulfomethyl
Ref. Hoeprich, P. D.: The Polymyxins. Med Clin N Amer, 54:1257, 1970.

743. EFFECTIVENESS OF GRISEOFULVIN THERAPY IN THE TREATMENT OF:
A. Tinea pedis
B. Tinea capitis
Ref. Goldman, L.: Griseofulvin. Med Clin N Amer, 54:1339, 1970.

744. INCIDENCE OF RASH AMONG PATIENTS RECEIVING:
A. Ampicillin
B. Ampicillin and allopurinol
Ref. Boston Collaborative Drug Surveillance Program. Excess of Ampicil-
lin Rashes Associated with Allopurinol or Hyperuricemia. New Eng
J Med. 286:505, 1972.

745. ANTIBACTERIAL POTENCY OF:
A. Desacetylcephalothin
B. Cephalothin
Ref. Saslaw, S.: Cephalosporins. Med Clin N Amer, 54:1217, 1970.

746. THE PERCENTAGE OF AN ABSORBED DOSE OF CEPHALOGLYCIN
EXCRETED IN THE URINE AS:
A. Cephaloglycin
B. Desacetylcephaloglycin
Ref. Saslaw, S.: Cephalosporins. Med Clin N Amer, 54:1217, 1970.

747. STABILITY OF CEPHALEXIN AT ROOM TEMPERATURE IN FLUIDS OF:
A. pH4
B. pH7
Ref. Griffith, R. S., Black, H. R., Cephalexin. Med Clin N Amer,
54:1229, 1970.

748. RISE IN B. U. N. AMONG PATIENTS RECEIVING:
A. Tetracycline
B. Tetracycline and diuretics
Ref. Boston Collaborative Drug Surveillance Program. Tetracycline and
Drug Attributed Rises in Blood Urea Nitrogen. JAMA, 220:377, 1972.

749. THE SERUM HALF-LIFE OF PENICILLIN IN:
A. Anuric patients with normal hepatic function
B. Anuric patients with decreased hepatic function
Ref. Kunin, C. M., Finland, M., J Clin Invest, 38:1509, 1959.

750. AMOUNT OF INJECTED PENICILLIN EXCRETED BY:
A. Glomerular filtration
B. Tubular secretion
Ref. Fishman, L. S., Hewitt, W. L.: The Natural Penicillins.
Med Clin N America, 54:1081, 1970.

751. PERCENTAGE OF ADMINISTERED DOSE RECOVERED IN THE URINE
8 HOURS AFTER ADMINISTRATION:
A. Phenoxymethyl penicillin
B. Benzylpenicillin
Ref. Sabath, L. D., Phenoxymethyl Penicillin (Penicillin V) and
Phenethecillin. Med Clin N Amer, 54:1101, 1970.

752.   THE RENAL CLEARANCE OF:
       A. Creatinine
       B. Methicillin
       Ref. Gilbert, D. N., Sanford, J. P.: Methicillin: Critical Appraisal
       After a Decade of Experience. Med Clin N Amer, 54:1113, 1970.

753.   MORTALITY RATE IN PATIENTS WITH STAPHYLOCOCCAL
       BACTEREMIA TREATED WITH:
       A. Methicillin
       B. Oxacillin
       Ref. Gilbert, D. N., Sanford, J. P.: Methicillin: Critical Appraisal
       After a Decade of Experience. Med Clin N Amer, 54:1113, 1970.

754.   PLASMA CLEARANCE OF GENTAMICIN:
       A. Normal renal function
       B. Impaired renal function
       Ref. Cutler, R. E., Gyselynck, A. M., Fleet, W. P., et al: Correlation
       of Serum Creatinine Concentration and Gentamicin Half-Life. JAMA,
       219, 1037, 1972.

755.   SERUM HALF-LIFE OF CHLORTETRACYCLINE:
       A. Patient with normal renal function
       B. Patient with serum creatinine of 5mg/100 ml
       Ref. Kunin, C. M., Finland, M.: Persistence of Antibiotics in Blood of
       Patients with Acute Renal Failure; 1. Tetracycline and Chlortetracycline.
       J Clin Invest, 38:1487, 1959.

756.   PRICE TO THE PATIENT OF 10 DAYS THERAPY WITH:
       A. Dicloxacillin (500 mg per day)
       B. Nafcillin (1 gm per day)
       Ref. Handbook of Antimicrobial Therapy. The Medical Letter, 14:51, 1972.

757.   STABILITY OF:
       A. Oxacillin in NaCl 0.9% solution
       B. Kanamycin in NaCl 0.9% solution
       Ref. Handbook of Antimicrobial Therapy. The Medical Letter, 14:34, 1972.

758.   SYSTEMIC ABSORPTION OF NEOMYCIN ADMINISTERED BY:
       A. The oral route
       B. Enema
       Ref. Breen, K. J., Bryant, R. E., Levinson, J. D., Schenker, S.:
       Neomycin Absorption in Man. Ann Int Med, 76:211, 1972.

759.   DURATION OF THERAPY WITH:
       A. Penicillin in acute uncomplicated pneumococcal pneumonia
       B. Erythromycin in severe mycoplasma pneumoniae pneumonia
       Ref. Handbook of Antimicrobial Therapy. The Medical Letter, 14:26, 1972.

760.   ZONE OF INHIBITION OF A SENSITIVE ORGANISM AROUND AN
       AMINOGLYCOSIDE ANTIBIOTIC DISC INCUBATED:
       A. In room air
       B. In 5% CO_2
       Ref. Ericsson, H. M., Sherris, J. C.: Antibiotic Sensitivity Testing.
       Acta Pathol Microbiol Scand, S127, 1971.

761.   RENAL CLEARANCE OF:
       A. Oxytetracycline
       B. Doxycycline
       Ref. The Medical Letter, 14:4, 1972.

762.   RENAL CLEARANCE OF:
A.   Tetracycline HCl
B.   Tetracycline phosphate complex
Ref. The Medical Letter, 14:4, 1972.

763.   TRAUMATIC JOINT FLUID CONCENTRATION/SERUM CONCENTRATION
RATIO OF:
A.   Ampicillin two hours after administration of 500 mg of ampicillin by
the oral route
B.   Kanamycin two hours after administration of 15 mg/kg body weight by
the intramuscular route
Ref. Baciocco, E. A., Iles, R. L.: Ampicillin and Kanamycin Concentration
in Joint Fluid. Clin Pharmacol Ther, 12:858, 1971.

764.   SERUM NITROFURANTOIN LEVELS TWO HOURS AFTER ORAL
ADMINISTRATION OF 100 mgm OF:
A.   Nitrofurantoin - normal person
B.   Nitrofurantoin - patient with renal insufficiency
Ref. Felts, J. H., Hayes, D. M., Gergen, J. A., et al: Neural, Hema-
tologic and Bacteriologic Effects of Nitrofurantoin in Renal Insufficiency.
Amer J Med, 51, 331, 1971.

765.   URINARY CONCENTRATION OF NITROFURANTOIN 6 HOURS AFTER
ORAL ADMINISTRATION OF 100 mgm OF:
A.   Nitrofurantoin - normal person
B.   Nitrofurantoin - patient with renal insufficiency
Ref. Felts, J. H., Hayes, D. M., Gergen, J. A., et al: Neural, Hema-
tologic and Bacteriologic Effects of Nitrofurantoin in Renal Insufficiency.
Amer J Med, 51:331, 1971.

766.   CONCENTRATION OF:
A.   Gentamicin in human bile
B.   Ampicillin in human bile
Ref. Smithvias, T., Hyams, P. J., Rahal, J. J.: Gentamicin and
Ampicillin in Human Bile. J Inf Dis, 124(S):106, 1971.

767.   AGAINST ENTEROCOCCI, H. INFLUENZAE, AND ENTEROBACTER
AEROGENES, WHICH OF THE FOLLOWING IS GREATER?:
A.   Activity of cephalexin
B.   Activity of ampicillin
Ref. Kunin, C. M., Finkelberg, Z.: Oral Cephalexin and Ampicillin:
Antimicrobial Activity Recovery in Urine and Persistence in Blood of
Uremic Patients. Ann Intern Med, 72:349, 1970.

768.   FOLLOWING ORAL ADMINISTRATION OF EQUAL AMOUNTS OF EACH
ANTIBIOTIC:
A.   Urinary concentration of cephaloglycin
B.   Urinary concentration of cephaloridine
Ref. Perkins, R. L., Glontz, G. E., Saslaw, S.: Cephaloglycin:
Crossover Absorption Studies and Clinical Evaluation. Clin Pharmacol
Ther, 10:244, 1969.

769.   A.   Minimum inhibitory concentration (MIC) of colistin for Serratia
marcescens
B.   MIC of colistin for Klebsiella sp.
Ref. Greenup, P., Blazevic, D. J.: Antibiotic Susceptibilities of Serratia
Marcescens and Enterobacter Liquefaciens. Appl Microbiol, 22:309, 1971.

770.   SERUM T$\frac{1}{2}$ OF:
A. Ampicillin in mouse serum
B. Epicillin in mouse serum
Ref. Godebusch, H., Miraglia, G., Pansy, F., Et al: Epicillin:
Experimental Chemotherapy, Pharmacodynamics, and Susceptibility
Testing. Inf and Imm, 4:50, 1971.

771.   COMPARE THE INCIDENCE OF SUBDURAL EFFUSIONS AMONG
CHILDREN WITH H. INFLUENZA MENINGITIS:
A. Treated with ampicillin
B. Treated with chloramphenicol
Ref. Schulkind, M. L., Altemeier, W. A., Ayoub, E. M.: A Comparison
of Ampicillin and Chloramphenicol Therapy in Hemophilus Influenzae
Meningitis. Pediatrics, 48:411, 1971.

772.   SENSITIVITY OF:
A. Stable L forms of P. aeruginosa to gentamicin
B. Bacterial form of P. aeruginosa to gentamicin
Ref. Hubert, E. G., Potter, C. S., Hensley, T. J., et al: L Forms of
Pseudomonas Aeruginosa. Inf and Imm, 4:60, 1971.

773.   RATIO OF AVERAGE CONCENTRATION OF TETRACYCLINE IN:
A. Lung to average concentration of tetracycline in serum
B. Muscle to average concentration of tetracycline in serum
Ref. Racz, G.: Tissue Concentrations of Antibiotic Following Oral
Doses of Tetracycline Phosphate Complex. Current Therap Res, 13:553,
1971.

774.   RATE OF UNTOWARD EFFECTS SEVERE ENOUGH TO REQUIRE
DISCONTINUATION OF THERAPY WITH:
A. Nitrofurantoin in hospitalized patients
B. Sulfisoxazole in hospitalized patients
Ref. Koch-Wesser, J., Sidel, V. W., Dexter, M., et al: Adverse
Reactions to Sulfisoxazole, Sulfamethoxazole and Nitrofurantoin.
Arch Intern Med, 128:399, 1971.

775.   THE PERCENTAGE OF STRAINS OF PROTEUS SPECIES, ISOLATED IN
GENERAL HOSPITAL, SENSITIVE TO CONCENTRATIONS OF:
A. Carbenicillin which could be achieved by recommended doses
B. Ampicillin which could be achieved by recommended doses
Ref. Adler, J., Burke, J. P., Martin, D. F., Finland, M.: Proteus
Infections in a General Hospital. Ann Intern Med, 75:517-530, 1971.

776.   RENAL:
A. Lymph concentrations of gentamicin
B. Urine concentrations of gentamicin
Ref. Chisholm, G. M.: Distribution and Dosage of Antibacterial Agents
in Patients with Normal and Impaired Renal Function. Med J Aust,
1:supp, 25-29, 1970.

777.   ANTIBACTERIAL ACTIVITY OF ERYTHROMYCIN AT:
A. Acid pH
B. Alkaline pH
Ref. Zinner, S. H., Sobath, L. D., Casey, J. I., Finland, M.:
Erythromycin and Alkalinisation of the Urine in the Treatment of Urinary
Tract Infections due to Gram-Negative Bacilli. Lancet, 1:1267, 1971.

778. SENSITIVITY OF P. AERUGINOSA TO:
A. Sulfisoxazole
B. Sulfamethoxazole
Ref. Dalton, A. C. , Meyers, S. D. : Sensitivity of Pseudomonas Aeruginosa
to Sulfamethoxazole. Amer J Clin Path, 56:371, 1971.

779. MINIMUM INHIBITORY CONCENTRATION OF:
A. Penicillin G for most strains of N. gonorrhoeae
B. Streptomycin for most strains of N. gonorrhoeae
Ref. Cave, V. G. , Hurdle, E. S. , Catelli, A. R. : Sensitivity of Neisseria
Gonorrhoea to Penicillin and Other Drugs. New York J Med, 70:844, 1970.

780. ABOLITION OF CARRIER STATE FOR C. DIPHTHERIAE AFTER:
A. 8 days of treatment with erythromycin estolate 250 mgm qid
B. Injection of 1. 2 million units of benzathine penicillin
Ref. McCloskey, R. V. , Eller, J. J. , Green, M. , et al: The 1970
Epidemic of Diphtheria in San Antonio. Ann Intern Med, 75:495-503, 1971.

781. URINARY LEVELS OF CARBENICILLIN 6 HOURS AFTER:
A. Oral ingestion of 500 mg of carbenicillin
B. Intramuscular administration of 500 mg of carbenicillin
Ref. Acred, P. , Brown, D. M. , Knudsen, E. T. , et al: New Semi-
Synthetic Penicillin Active Against Pseudomonas Pyocyanea. Nature,
215:25, 1967.

782. SERUM LEVELS OF CARBENICILLIN AFTER ADMINISTRATION OF 5g
OF DRUG BY:
A. Rapid intravenous infusion
B. Rapid intravenous infusion 1 hour after oral administration of 0.5 g
probenecid
Ref. Bodey, G. P. , Rodriquez, V. , Stewart, O. : Clinical Pharmacologic
Studies of Carbenicillin. Am J Med Sci, 257:185, 1969.

783. EFFECTIVENESS OF HUMAN GAMMA GLOBULIN IN PREVENTING:
A. Secondary cases of infectious hepatitis
B. Post-transfusion hepatitis
Ref. Chalmers, T. C. , Alter, H. J. : Management of the Asymptomatic
Carrier of the Hepatitis-Associated (Australia) Antigen. New Eng J Med,
285:613, 1971.

784. MINIMUM INHIBITORY CONCENTRATION OF:
A. Carbenicillin against indole positive proteus species
B. Ampicillin against indole positive proteus species
Ref. Acred, P. , Brown, D. M. , Knudsen, E. T. , et al: New Semi-
Synthetic Penicillin Active Against Pseudomonas Pyocyanea. Nature,
215:25, 1967.

EACH SET OF LETTERED HEADINGS IS FOLLOWED BY A NUMBERED
LIST OF WORDS OR PHRASES. ANSWER:
A. If the word or phrase is associated with A only
B. If the word or phrase is associated with B only
C. If the word or phrase is associated with A and B
D. If the word or phrase is associated with neither A nor B

A. Sodium colistimethate
B. Polymyxin B sulfate
C. Both
D. Neither

785. ___ Effective against Proteus
786. ___ Effective against Providencia sp.
787. ___ Local pain frequent on injection
788. ___ High antibacterial concentration in urine
789. ___ Nephrotoxic
790. ___ Neurotoxic
      Ref. Goodwin, N. J., Colistin and Sodium Colistimethate. Med Clin N
      Amer, 54:1273, 1970.

A. Primarily bacteriostatic
B. Primarily bactericidal
C. Both
D. Neither

791. ___ Chloramphenicol
792. ___ Vancomycin
793. ___ Penicillin
794. ___ Cephalothin
795. ___ Amphotericin B
796. ___ Streptomycin
797. ___ Nalidixic acid
798. ___ Erythromycin
      Ref. Fekety, F. R., Allen, J. C., Cluff, L. E.: Management of Infectious
      Diseases in The Principles and Practice of Medicine, 17th Ed, Chap 67,
      Appleton-Century-Crofts, New York, 1968, pp. 671-686.

A. Cephalothin
B. Cephaloridine
C. Both
D. Neither

799. ___ Excreted unchanged in the urine
800. ___ Excreted predominantly by glomerular filtration
801. ___ Excreted by both glomerular filtration and tubular secretion
802. ___ Useful for treatment of urinary infections
803. ___ Does produce therapeutic serum levels
      Ref. Griffith, R. S., Black, H. R.: Blood, Urine, and Tissue Concentrations
      of the Cephalosporin Antibiotics in Normal Subjects. Postgrad Med J,
      47:32, 1971.

A. Gram positive bacteremia
B. Gram negative bacteremia
C. Both
D. Neither

804. ___ Positive Limulus test
805. ___ Intravascular coagulation
806. ___ Hypofibrinogenemia
807. ___ Constant reduction of serum complement
808. ___ Endotoxemia constant
Ref. Levin, J., Poore, T. E., Young, N. S., et al: Gram Negative Sepsis: Detection of Endotoxemia with the Limulus Test. Ann Int Med, 76:1, 1971.

A. Cloxacillin
B. Dicloxacillin
C. Both
D. Neither

809. ___ Effective at low concentrations against Group A streptococci
810. ___ As effective as penicillin G against D. pneumoniae
811. ___ Renal clearance approximately 160 ml/min/M^2
812. ___ Good activity against H. influenzae
813. ___ Highest serum concentrations after oral administration
814. ___ Cross the placental barrier
Ref. Marcy, S. M., Klein, J. O.: The Isoxazolyl Penicillins. Med Clin N Amer, 54:1127, 1970.

IN THE FOLLOWING, CHOOSE:
A. If 1, 2 and 3 are correct
B. If 1 and 3 are correct
C. If 2 and 4 are correct
D. If only 4 is correct
E. If all four are correct

815. RESISTANCE TO LINCOMYCIN AND ERYTHROMYCIN HAS BEEN REPORTED AMONG THE FOLLOWING SPECIES OF BACTERIA:
1. E. coli
2. Group A streptococci
3. P. aeruginosa
4. D. pneumoniae
Ref. Dixon, J. M. S., Lipinski, A. E.: Resistance of Group A Beta Hemolytic Streptococci to Lincomycin and Erythromycin. Antimicrob Ag Chemother, 1:333, 1972.

816. WHICH OF THE FOLLOWING DEMONSTRATE SYNERGISM WITH PENICILLIN AGAINST ENTEROCOCCI?:
1. Cephalothin
2. Erythromycin
3. EDTA
4. Tetracycline
Ref. Moellering, R. C., Wennersten, C., Weinberg, A. N.: Studies on Antibiotic Synergism Against Enterococci. Bacteriologic Studies. J Lab Clin Med, 77:821, 1971.

817.   IN PATIENTS WITH NORMAL RENAL FUNCTION AND DOCUMENTED
       ALLERGY TO PENICILLIN, CEPHALORIDINE IS RECOMMENDED FOR
       THE TREATMENT OF MENINGITIS DUE TO:
       1. Hemophilus
       2. Pneumococcus
       3. Meningococcus
       4. Streptococcus
       Ref. Lerner, P. I.: Penetration of Cephaloridine into Cerebrospinal Fluid.
       Amer J Med Sci, 262:321, 1971.

818.   THE FOLLOWING DRUGS ARE EFFECTIVE IN TREATMENT OF ACUTE
       BRUCELLOSIS:
       1. Chloramphenicol
       2. Tetracycline
       3. Trimethoprim-sulfamethoxazole
       4. Streptomycin
       Ref. Giunchi, G., deRosa, F., Babiani, F.: Trimethoprim-Sulfamethoxa-
       zole Combination in the Treatment of Acute Human Brucellosis. Chemother,
       16:332, 1971.

819.   VANCOMYCIN IS BACTERICIDAL FOR:
       1. Salmonella sp.
       2. Staphylococci sp.
       3. M. tuberculosis
       4. Clostridia sp.
       Ref. Riley, H. D., Jr.: Vancomycin and Novobiocin. Med Clin N Amer,
       54:1277, 1970.

820.   PROPHYLACTIC USE OF EITHER PENICILLIN OR AMPICILLIN FOR 5
       DAYS AFTER CLOSED HEART SURGERY AFFECTS THE CHARACTER OF
       POST OPERATIVE INFECTIONS IN WHICH OF THE FOLLOWING WAYS?:
       1. Post operative infections are more likely to be caused by Gram
           negative rather than Gram positive organisms
       2. Patients receiving antibiotics have more days of fever than those not
           receiving antibiotics
       3. Most infecting organisms are resistant to the prophylactically
           administered antibiotics
       4. The total number of infections is reduced in the group receiving
           prophylactic antibiotic therapy
       Ref. Sallam, I. A., Sammon, A., McGeachie, J., et al: Prophylactic
       Antibiotics in Closed Heart Surgery. Chest, 60:252, 1971.

821.   WHICH OF THE FOLLOWING ANTIBIOTICS SHOW A SYNERGISTIC
       EFFECT WITH PENICILLIN AGAINST ENTEROCOCCI IN VITRO?:
       1. Chloramphenicol
       2. Cycloserine
       3. Erythromycin
       4. Vancomycin
       Ref. Moellering, R. C., Weinberg, A.: Studies on Antibiotic Synergism
       Against Enterococci. J Clin Invest, 50:2580, 1971.

822.   IN WHICH OF THE FOLLOWING DISEASES IS TREATMENT WITH
       STREPTOMYCIN ALONE BOTH EFFECTIVE AND JUSTIFIABLE?:
       1. Enterococcal endocarditis
       2. Brucellosis
       3. Tuberculosis
       4. Tularemia
       Ref. Martin, W. J.: The Present Status of Streptomycin in Antimicrobial
       Therapy. Med Clin N Amer, 54:1161, 1970.

823. SIDE EFFECTS OF TETRACYCLINE THERAPY INCLUDE:
      1. Onycholysis
      2. Nephrogenic diabetes insipidus
      3. Increased intracranial pressure
      4. Simulated lupus erythematosus
      Ref. Ory, E. M.: The Tetracyclines. Med Clin N Amer, 54:1173, 1970.

824. CHLORAMPHENICOL WOULD BE SUPERIOR TO OTHER DRUGS AND
      THEREFORE THE DRUG OF CHOICE IN THE TREATMENT OF:
      1. Enteric fever
      2. Tularemia
      3. Plague
      4. Typhoid fever
      Ref. Snyder, M. J., Woodward, T. E.: The Clinical Use of Chloramphenicol.
      Med Clin N Amer, 54:1193, 1970.

825. WHICH OF THE FOLLOWING ARE RECOGNIZED SIDE EFFECTS OF
      PIPERAZINE THERAPY?:
      1. Allergic rashes
      2. Nausea and vomiting
      3, Cerebellar ataxia
      4. Femoral head necrosis
      Ref. Parsons, A. C.: Piperazine Neurotoxicity: "Worm Wobble."
      Br Med J, 4:792, 1971.

826. THE METHICILLIN CONCENTRATION OF WHICH OF THE FOLLOWING
      FLUIDS WOULD BE ESSENTIALLY EQUAL TO A SIMULTANEOUSLY
      OBTAINED SERUM LEVEL IN A NORMAL PERSON?:
      1. Pleural fluid
      2. Pericardial fluid
      3. Ascitic fluid
      4. Cerebrospinal fluid
      Ref. White, A., Varga, D. T.: Antistaphylococcal Activity of Sodium
      Methicillin. Arch Intern Med, 108:671, 1961.

827. WHICH OF THE FOLLOWING ANTIBIOTICS ARE INCOMPATIBLE WITH
      NaCl 0.9% SOLUTION?:
      1. Erythromycin lactobionate
      2. Nafcillin
      3. Amphotericin B
      4. Gentamicin
      Ref. Handbook of Antimicrobial Therapy. The Medical Letter, 14:35, 1972.

828. THE TOXIC EFFECTS OF AMPHOTERICIN B ON THE KIDNEY INCLUDE:
      1.. Hypokalemia
      2. Tubular degeneration
      3. Renal tubular acidosis
      4. Renal potassium wasting
      Ref. Gouge, T. H., Andriole, V. T.: An Experimental Model of
      Amphotericin B Nephrotoxicity with Renal Tubular Acidosis. J Lab Clin
      Med, 78:713, 1971.

829. WHICH OF THE FOLLOWING SEMI-SYNTHETIC PENICILLINS IS USEFUL
      IN TREATING INFECTIONS CAUSED BY PSEUDOMONAS AERUGINOSA?:
      1. Ampicillin
      2. Carbenicillin
      3. Dicloxacillin
      4. Epicillin
      Ref. Beck, J. E., Hubsher, J. A., Caloza, D.: A Multi-Center Clinical
      Evaluation of Epicillin. Curr Therap Res, 13:530, 1971.

830.   THE CONCENTRATION OF WHICH OF THE FOLLOWING IONS GREATLY
        INFLUENCES THE MIC VALUE OF GENTAMICIN FOR P AERUGINOSA?:
        1. Potassium
        2. Magnesium
        3. Sulfate
        4. Calcium
        Ref. Medeiros, A. A. , O'Brien, T. F. , Wacker, W. E. L. , et al: Effect
        of Salt Concentration on the Apparent In-Vitro Susceptibility of
        Pseudomonas and Other Gram Negative Bacilli to Gentamicin.   J Inf Dis,
        124(S):59, 1971. Also Carache, P: Disscussion, Ibid, p. 68.

831.   THE RENAL EXCRETION OF GENTAMICIN INVOLVES THE FOLLOWING:
        1. Glomerular filtration
        2. Tubular reabsorption
        3. Tubular secretion
        4. Clearance exceeding that of inulin
        Ref. Gyselynck, A. M. , Forrey, A. , Cutler, R. : Pharmokinetics of
        Gentamicin: Distribution and Plasma and Renal Clearance. J Inf Dis,
        124(S):70, 1971.

832.   GENTAMICIN WOULD NOT BE CONSIDERED AN APPROPRIATE
        ANTIBIOTIC FOR TREATMENT OF INFECTION CAUSED BY WHICH OF
        THE FOLLOWING ORGANISMS?:
        1. Pneumococci
        2. Mima sp.
        3. Bacteroides sp.
        4. Providence sp.
        Ref. Second International Symposium on Gentamicin Discussion.
        J Inf Dis, 124(S):211, 1971.

833.   ADMINISTRATION OF PROBENECID INCREASES THE SERUM CONCEN-
        TRATION OF THE FOLLOWING ANTIBIOTICS:
        1. Carbenicillin
        2. Cephaloridine
        3. Penicillin
        4. Ampicillin
        Ref. The Medical Letter, 13:88, 1971.

834.   THE FOLLOWING DRUGS POTENTIATE THE ACTION OF COUMARIN IN
        MAN:
        1. Chloramphenicol
        2. Long-acting sulfonamides
        3. Neomycin
        4. Griseofulvin
        Ref. Koch-Weser, J. , Sellers, E. M. : Drug Interactions with Coumarin
        Anticoagulants. New Eng J Med, 285:547, 1971.

835.   GROWTH OF THE FOLLOWING ORGANISMS COULD BE EXPECTED TO
        BE INHIBITED BY CONCENTRATIONS OF CEPHALEXIN OBTAINED
        IN THE SERUM FOLLOWING RECOMMENDED DOSAGE
        SCHEDULES:
        1. "Enterococci"
        2. D. pneumoniae
        3. Pseudomonas aeruginosa
        4. Staphylococcus aureus
        Ref. Henning, C. , Kallings, L. O. , Lidman, K. , et al: Studies of
        Absorption, Excretion, Antibacterial and Clinical Effect of Cephalexin.
        Scand J Infect Dis, 2:131, 1970.

836.   OBSERVED COMPLICATIONS OF THE USE OF HYDROCORTISONE TO
       REDUCE SIDE EFFECTS OF AMPHOTERICIN B ADMINISTRATION
       INCLUDE:
       1. Cardiac enlargement
       2. Congestive heart failure
       3. Hypokalemic cardiopathy
       4. Decreased urinary potassium excretion
       Ref. Chung, D. K. , Koenig, M. G. : Reversible Cardiac Enlargement
       During Treatment with Amphotericin B and Hydrocortisone: Report of
       Three Cases. Amer Rev Resp Dis, 103:831, 1971.

837.   THE FOLLOWING ANTIBIOTICS ARE BACTERICIDAL FOR C.
       DIPHTHERIAE AT CONCENTRATIONS WHICH COULD BE OBTAINED BY
       RECOMMENDED ORAL DOSES:
       1. Ampicillin
       2. Clindamycin
       3. Rifampin
       4. Penicillin
       Ref. McCloskey, R. V. , Eller, J. J. , Green, M. , et al: The 1970
       Epidemic of Diphtheria in San Antonio. Ann Intern Med, 75:495-503.

       EACH GROUP OF ITEMS CONSISTS OF A LIST OF LETTERED
       HEADINGS FOLLOWED BY A LIST OF NUMBERED WORDS OR PHRASES.
       FOR EACH NUMBERED WORD OR PHRASE, SELECT THE ONE HEADING
       MOST CLOSELY RELATED TO IT:

       A. Positive Coombs' test
       B. Diarrhea
       C. Eighth cranial nerve damage
       D. Gastrointestinal disturbances
       E. Pulmonary infiltrates
       F. Neuromuscular blockade
       G. Hypothyroidism

838. ___ Lincomycin
839. ___ Nitrofurantoin
840. ___ Cephalothin
841. ___ Streptomycin
842. ___ Gentamicin
843. ___ Ethionamide
844. ___ Tetracyclines
       Ref. Handbook of Antimicrobial Therapy. The Medical Letter, 14:16, 1972.

       A. Penicillin G
       B. Penicillin G and streptomycin
       C. Oxacillin and kanamycin
       D. No antibiotics

845. ___ Surgery for heavily contaminated trauma
846. ___ Dental extraction patient with rheumatic heart disease
847. ___ Genitourinary procedure patient with rheumatic heart disease
848. ___ Extensively burned patients
849. ___ Closed heart surgery
       Ref. The Medical Letter, 14:25, 1972.

A. Chloramphenicol
B. Streptomycin
C. Penicillin
D. Carbenicillin
E. Gentamicin
F. Ampicillin
G. Kanamycin

850. ___ Shigellosis
851. ___ Typhoid fever
852. ___ Hospital-acquired E. coli sepsis
853. ___ E. coli sepsis acquired outside of hospital
854. ___ Hospital-acquired K. pneumoniae sepsis
855. ___ K. pneumoniae sepsis acquired outside of hospital
856. ___ Serratia sepsis
857. ___ Providencia sepsis
858. ___ Pasturella multocida wound infection
Ref. Handbook of Antimicrobial Therapy. The Medical Letter, 14:12, 1972.

A. Penicillins and cephalosporins
B. Chloramphenicol
C. Tetracycline
D. Streptomycin
E. Polymycin
F. Nalidixic acid
G. Rifampin

859. ___ Blocks DNA synthesis
860. ___ Blocks RNA synthesis
861. ___ Blocks binding of t-RNA-amino acid complex to ribosome
862. ___ Interferes with function of m-RNA
863. ___ Blocks transfer of amino acids into amino acid chain
864. ___ Disrupt cytoplasmic membrane
865. ___ Stops cross-linking of linear peptide strands during cell wall synthesis
Ref. Lorian, V.: The Mode of Action of Antibiotics on Gram-Negative Bacilli. Ann Intern Med, 128:623, 1971.

A. Sternoclavicular joint involved
B. Intra-articular antibiotics necessary
C. Intra-articular antibiotics usually not required

866. ___ Bacteroides sp. arthritis
867. ___ Septic arthritis complicating rheumatoid arthritis
868. ___ Group A βHemolytic streptococcal arthritis
869. ___ Pseudomonas aeruginosa arthritis
Ref. Tindel, J. R., Crowder, J. G.: Septic Arthritis Due to Pseudomonas Aeruginosa. JAMA, 218:559, 1971.

A. Acidification of urine increases activity of antimicrobic against most sensitive strains of bacteria
B. Alkalinization of urine increases the activity of antimicrobic agent against most sensitive strains of bacteria
C. pH of urine has inconsistent effect or no effect on antibacterial activity

870. ___ Chlortetracycline
871. ___ Methenamine mandelate
872. ___ Gentamicin
873. ___ Chloramphenicol
874. ___ Cephaloridine
875. ___ Ampicillin
876. ___ Erythromycin
877. ___ Kanamycin
878. ___ Nitrofurantoin
Ref. Lan, G. R., Levin, S.: Diagnosis and Treatment of Urinary Tract Infections. Med Clin N Amer, 55:1439, 1971.

A. Tetracycline hydrochloride
B. Methacycline
C. Oxytetracycline
D. Minocycline

879. ___ Renal clearance = 90 ml/min
880. ___ Renal clearance = 65 ml/min
881. ___ Renal clearance = 31 ml/min
882. ___ Renal clearance - 9 ml/min
Ref. The Medical Letter, 14:4, 1972.

A. Dapsone
B. Acedapsone
C. Clofazimine
D. Rifampicin

883. ___ Repository sulfone preparation
884. ___ Standard dose in man is 50 to 100 mg daily
885. ___ Red pigmentation of the skin
886. ___ Rapid bactericidal capacity
Ref. Shepard. C. C.: The First Decade in Experimental Leprosy. Bull Wld Hlth Org, 44:821, 1971.

A. Appendix
B. Gallbladder
C. Kidney
D. Spleen

Organ	Ratio of average tissue concentration of tetracycline to average serum concentration of tetracycline
887. ___ ---	0.4
888. ___ ---	2.0
889. ___ ---	3.0
890. ___ ---	4.2

Ref. Racz, G.: Tissue Concentrations of Antibiotic Following Oral Dose of Tetracycline Phosphate Complex. Current Therap Res, 13:553, 1971.

      A. Kirby-Bauer technique
      B. Pour plate technique
      C. Hemoglobin reduction technique

891. ___ Swab used to inoculate standard number of bacteria
892. ___ Can be interpreted in 4 hours
893. ___ Requires 2 hour incubation period prior to inoculation of sensitivity plates
Ref. Melia, J. L., Cook, E. L., White, R. S.: Rapid Antibiotic Sensitivity Testing Using Zone Size Methodology. Amer J Clin Path, 56:59, 1971.

      A. Penicillin
      B. Cephalothin
      C. Chloramphenicol
      D. Lincomycin
      E. Gentamicin

ALL QUESTIONS REFER TO PATIENTS WITH RENAL INSUFFICIENCY:

894. ___ Metabolic encephalopathy with convulsions
895. ___ No known increase in side effects
896. ___ Depressed erythropoiesis
897. ___ Nephrotoxicity
898. ___ Suprainfection with resistant organisms
Ref. Bulger, R. J., Petersdorf, R. G.: Antimicrobial Therapy in Patients with Renal Insufficiency. Postgrad Med J, 47:160, 1970.

QUESTIONS 899-903 RELATE TO THE LENGTH OF TREAT-
MENT WITH CEPHALOTHIN OF VARIOUS INFECTIONS CAUSED BY
S. AUREUS:

      A. Endocarditis - artificial valve
      B. Endocarditis
      C. Pneumonia
      D. Septic arthritis
      E. Pyelonephritis

899. ___ Two weeks per course
900. ___ Twelve weeks
901. ___ Four to eight weeks
902. ___ Seven days after the temperature returns
903. ___ Six weeks
Ref. Smith, I. M.: Cephalosporin Therapy of Staphylococcal Infections in Adults. Postgrad Med J, 47:78, 1971.

    A. Penicillin
    B. Tetracyclines
    C. Vancomycin
    D. Novobiocin
    E. Chloramphenicol

904. ___ Reversible bone marrow depression
905. ___ Yellow serum pigment
906. ___ Acute hepatic necrosis
907. ___ Thrombophlebitis
908. ___ Anaphylaxis

Ref. Fekety, F. R. , Allen, J. C. , Cluff, L. E.: Management of
Infectious Diseases in The Principles and Practice of Medicine,
17th Ed, Chap 67, Appleton-Century-Crofts, New York, 1968, pp. 671-686.

FOR EACH OF THE FOLLOWING MULTIPLE CHOICE QUESTIONS,
SELECT THE ONE MOST APPROPRIATE ANSWER:

909.   AMEBIC PERICARDITIS IS USUALLY ASSOCIATED WITH ALL OF THE
       FOLLOWING, EXCEPT:
       A. Liver abscess
       B. Constrictive pericarditis
       C. Positive stool for amebae
       D. Serum amebic hemagglutinins
       E. Sterile pus in liver
       Ref. Heller, R. F. , Gorbach, S. L. , Tatooles, C. J. , et al: Amebic
       Pericarditis. JAMA, 220:988, 1972.

910.   WHICH OF THE FOLLOWING SYNDROMES IS MOST SUGGESTIVE OF
       TRICHINOSIS?:
       A. Leukocytosis with eosinophilia
       B. Leukopenia, eosinophilia, fever
       C. Myalgia, facial edema, fever
       D. Malaise, headache, diaphoresis
       E. Chills, nausea, leukopenia
       Ref. Wand, M. , Lyman, D. : Trichinosis from Bear Meat. JAMA,
       220:245, 1972.

911.   SCRUB TYPHUS (INFECTION BY R. TSUTSUGAMUSHI) IS ACQUIRED BY
       NUMBERS OF UNITED STATES ARMED FORCES PERSONNEL IN
       VIETNAM.   THE MOST CHARACTERISTIC SKIN LESION OBSERVED
       DURING THESE OUTBREAKS IS:
       A. Grouped vesicles about the lips
       B. Pustules
       C. Macular rash on trunk
       D. Eschar
       E. Pox-like lesions
       Ref. Hazlett, D. R. : Scrub Typhus in Vietnam: Experience at the 8th
       Field Hospital. Milit Med, 135:31, 1970.

912.   WHICH OF THE FOLLOWING IS MOST COMMONLY OBSERVED IN
       ROCKY MOUNTAIN SPOTTED FEVER?:
       A. Parotitis
       B. Myocarditis
       C. Nuchal rigidity
       D. Skin ulceration
       E. Interstitial pneumonia
       Ref. Vianna, N. J. , Hinman, A. R. : Rocky Mountain Spotted Fever on
       Long Island. Amer J Med, 51:725, 1971.

913.   THE MOST COMMON MANIFESTATION OF PULMONARY DIROFILARIASIS
       IN MAN IS:
       A. Pleural effusion
       B. Coin lesion
       C. Pneumonia
       D. Lung abscess
       E. Bronchiectasis
       Ref. Navarette, A. R. : Pulmonary dirofilariasis. Chest, 61:51, 1972.

914.   THE MOST COMMON TYPE OF MALARIAL PARASITE CAUSING
       INFECTION IN VETERANS RETURNING TO THE U.S. FROM
       VIETNAM IS:
       A.   P. vivax
       B.   P. falciparum
       C.   P. malariae
       D.   P. ovale
       E.   Mixed infections
       Ref. Walzer, P.D., Dover, A.S., Schultz, M.G.: Malaria Surveillance
       in the United States and Puerto Rico. J Inf Dis, 125:194, 1972.

THE FOLLOWING QUESTIONS CONSIST OF PAIRS OF PHRASES
DESCRIBING CONDITIONS OR QUANTITIES WHICH MAY OR MAY NOT
VARY IN RELATION TO EACH OTHER.   ANSWER:
A.   If increase in the first is accompanied by increase in the second or
     decrease in the first is accompanied by decrease in the second
B.   If increase in the first is accompanied by decrease in the second or
     decrease in the first is accompanied by increase in the second
C.   If changes in the first are independent of changes in the second

915.   1.   Urine concentrating ability
       2.   Hydronephrosis
       Ref. Lehman, J.S., Farid, Z., Bassily, S., Kent, D.C.: Hydrone-
       phrosis, Bacteruria and Maximal Urine Concentration in Schistosomiasis.
       Ann Intern Med, 75:49, 1971.

916.   1.   Deformability of red cell
       2.   Number of red cells infested with plasmodia
       Ref. Miller, L.H., Usami, S., Chien, S.: Alteration in the rheologic
       properties of Plasmodium knowlesi - Infected Red Cells.   A Possible
       Mechanism for Capillary Obstruction. J Clin Invest, 50:1451, 1971.

917.   1.   Serum titer of Sabin-Feldman dye test toxoplasmosis antibody
       2.   Lymphocyte transformation to T. gondii antigen
       Ref. Krahenbuhl, J.L., Gaines, J.D., Remington, J.S.: Lymphocyte
       Transformation in Human Toxoplasmosis. J Inf Dis, 125:283, 1972.

ANSWER THE FOLLOWING QUESTIONS ACCORDING TO THE KEY
BELOW:
A.   If choice A is greater than choice B
B.   If choice B is greater than choice A
C.   If A and B are equal or nearly equal

918.   THE NUMBERS OF PATIENTS TREATED WITH PYRANTEL PAMOATE
       WHO ARE CURED OF INFESTATION WITH:
       A.   Ascaris lumbricoides
       B.   Trichuris trichuria
       Ref. Villarejos, V.M.: Experience with Anthelminthic Pyrantel Pamoate.
       Am J Trop Med Hyg, 20:842, 1971.

919.   ASSESS THE SENSITIVITY OF THE FOLLOWING TESTS IN THE
       DIAGNOSIS OF HUMAN HYDATID DISEASE:
       A.   Indirect hemagglutination test
       B.   Complement fixation test
       Ref. Miller, C.W., Ruppaner, R., Schwabe, C.W.: Hydatid Disease
       in California. Am J Trop Med Hyg, 20:904, 1971.

920.   SCHIZONTOCIDAL ACTIVITY OF:
        A. Quinine
        B. Sulphones
        Ref. Peters, W.: Chemotherapeutic Agents in Tropical Diseases in
        Recent Advances in Pharmacology, Chap 19, Ed by Robson, J. M., Stacey,
        R. S.: Little, Brown & Co., Boston, 1968, pp. 503-537.

        EACH SET OF LETTERED HEADINGS IS FOLLOWED BY A NUMBERED
        LIST OF WORDS OR PHRASES. ANSWER:
        A. If the word or phrase is associated with A only
        B. If the word or phrase is associated with B only
        C. If the word or phrase is associated with A and B
        D. If the word or phrase is associated with neither A nor B

        A. Malaria due to P. falciparum
        B. Malaria due to P. vivax
        C. Both
        D. Neither

921.   ___ Infection usually manifest within 1 month after leaving endemic area
922.   ___ First attack may produce daily irregular nondiagnostic fever
923.   ___ Infection may not be manifest for a year or more after leaving endemic
            area
924.   ___ Fever, chills, headache, myalgia
925.   ___ Characteristic physical findings
926.   ___ Elevated SGOT
927.   ___ Drug resistance
928.   ___ Hemolysis
929.   ___ Sausage-shaped gametocytes
        Ref. Heineman, H. S.: The Clinical Syndrome of Malaria in the United
        States. Arch Intern Med, 129:607, 1972.

        IN THE FOLLOWING QUESTIONS, CHOOSE:
        A. If 1, 2 and 3 are correct
        B. If 1 and 3 are correct
        C. If 2 and 4 are correct
        D. If only 4 is correct
        E. If all four are correct

930.   THE FOLLOWING DRUGS ARE EFFECTIVE IN PRODUCING RADICAL
        CURE OF CHLOROQUINE-RESISTANT P. FALCIPARUM MALARIA:
        1. Sulfones
        2. Tetracycline
        3. Trimethoprim-sulfamethoxazole
        4. Pyrimethamine-sulphormethoxine
        Ref. Colwell, E. J., Hickman, R. L., Kosakal, S.: Tetracycline
        Treatment of Chloroquine Resistant Falciparum Malaria in Thailand.
        JAMA, 220:684, 1972.

931.   OVER 99% OF THE CASES OF MALARIA SEEN IN AMERICANS
        RETURNING FROM SOUTHEAST ASIA ARE CAUSED BY:
        1. Plasmodium falciparum
        2. Plasmodium ovale
        3. Plasmodium vivax
        4. Plasmodium knowelesii
        Ref. Deller, J. J.: Malaria - Again a Diagnostic Consideration. A. F. P.,
        5:68, 1972.

932. WHICH OF THE FOLLOWING IS A KNOWN SOURCE OF INFECTION WITH TOXOPLASMA GONDII?:
1. Ticks
2. Poorly cooked meat
3. Lice
4. Cat feces
Ref. Kimball, A. C., Kean, B. H., Fuchs, F.: The Role of Toxoplasmosis in Abortion. Am J Obst Gynec, 111:219, 1971.

933. WHICH OF THE FOLLOWING ARE CHARACTERISTIC OF HUMAN GIARDIOSIS?:
1. Normal sigmoidoscopy
2. Bloody stools
3. Diarrhea
4. Chills
Ref. Babb, R. R., Peck, O. C., Vescia, F. G.: Giardiosis: A Cause of Travelers' Diarrhea. JAMA, 217:1359, 1971.

934. DRUGS EFFECTIVE IN THE TREATMENT OF GIARDIA LAMBLIA INFESTATION ARE:
1. Metronidazole
2. Quinacrine
3. Furazolidine
4. Ampicillin
Ref. Babb, R. R., Peck, O. W., Vescia, F. G.: Giardiasis: A Cause of Travelers' Diarrhea. JAMA, 217:1359, 1971.

935. THE FOLLOWING SIGNS AND SYMPTOMS ARE OBSERVED IN MORE THAN 50% OF PATIENTS WITH ACUTE RENAL INSUFFICIENCY COMPLICATING FALCIPARUM MALARIA:
1. Hepatosplenomegaly
2. Chills
3. Jaundice
4. Obtunded mental state
Ref. Stone, W. J., Hanchett, J. E., Knepshield, J. H.: Acute Renal Insufficiency due to Falciparum Malaria. Arch Intern Med, 129:620, 1972.

936. THE CURRENTLY RECOMMENDED THERAPY FOR FALCIPARUM MALARIA INCLUDES THE FOLLOWING DRUGS:
1. Quinine sulfate
2. Pyrimethamine
3. Dapsone
4. Chloroquin
Ref. Stone, W. J., Hanchett, J. E., Knepshield, J. H.: Acute Renal Insufficiency due to Falciparum Malaria. Arch Int Med, 129:620, 1972.

937. SYSTEMIC AMEBICIDES ACTIVE AGAINST AMEBAE IN THE LIVER INCLUDE:
1. Metronidazole
2. Emetine
3. Chloroquine
4. Tetracycline
Ref. Peters, W.: Chemotherapeutic Agents in Tropical Diseases in Recent Advances in Pharmacology, Chap 19, Ed. Robson, J. M., Stacv, R. S., Little, Brown & Co., Boston, 1968, pp. 503-537.

EACH GROUP OF ITEMS CONSISTS OF A LIST OF LETTERED
HEADINGS FOLLOWED BY A LIST OF NUMBERED WORDS OR PHRASES.
FOR EACH NUMBERED WORD OR PHRASE, SELECT THE ONE HEADING
MOST CLOSELY RELATED TO IT:

A. P. falciparum malaria
B. P. malariae malaria
C. P. ovale malaria
D. P. vivax malaria

938. ___ Incubation period may be as long as one month
939. ___ Daily or irregular fever
940. ___ Relapses many years after the first attack
941. ___ Relapses uncommon three years after first attack
942. ___ Most cases of transfusion malaria
Ref. Bruce-Chwatt, L. J.: Malaria. Brit Med J, 2:91, 1971.

A. Ascaris lumbricoides
B. Trichuris trichiura
C. Necator americanus
D. Strongyloides stercoralis
E. Taenia saginata
F. Schistosoma mansoni
G. Entamoebae histolytica

943. ___ No migratory phase through lung
944. ___ Largest of the intestinal nematodes of man
945. ___ Marked eosinophilia
946. ___ Penetration of exposed skin by larvae
947. ___ Cysticercosis
948. ___ Focal hepatic necrosis
949. ___ Hepatic cirrhosis
Ref. Miller, J. H., Abadie, S. H.: Common Intestinal Parasites of the
United States. South Med Bull, 59:11, 1971.

A. Metronidazole
B. Emetine
C. Sodium stibogluconate
D. Sulformethoxine and pyrimethamine

950. ___ Visceral leishmaniasis (Kala-azar)
951. ___ Dysenteric amebiasis
952. ___ Amebic hepatitis
953. ___ P. falciparum malaria
Ref. The Treatment of Tropical Diseases, Chap 2, 2nd Ed, Jopling, W. H.,
John Wright & Sons Ltd, Bristol, 1968.

A. Thiabendazole
B. Niridazole
C. Diethylcarbamazine citrate
D. Hydroxychlorobenzamide

954. ___ Ascariasis
955. ___ Hookworm infestation
956. ___ Filiariasis
957. ___ Bilharziasis
958. ___ Pinworm infestation
959. ___ Taeniasis
Ref. The Treatment of Tropical Diseases, Chap 1, 2nd Ed, Jopling W. H.,
John Wright & Sons Ltd, Bristol, 1968.

A. Piperazine citrate - drug of choice
B. Bephenium - drug of choice
C. Thiabendazole - drug of choice
D. No drug of choice
E. Hexylresorcinol

960. ___ Roundworm (Ascaris lumbricoides)
961. ___ Hookworm (Necator americanus)
962. ___ Whipworm (Trichuris trichiura)
963. ___ Pinworm (Enterobius vermicularis)
964. ___ Trichinosis (Trichinella spiralis)
965. ___ Visceral larva migrans
966. ___ Strongyloidiasis (Strongyloides stercoralis)
Ref. Handbook of Antimicrobial Therapy. The Medical Letter, 14:55, 1972.

FOR EACH OF THE FOLLOWING MULTIPLE CHOICE QUESTIONS,
SELECT THE ONE MOST APPROPRIATE ANSWER:

967.   IgM AND IgG ANTIBODIES ACTIVATE C1 WHICH IN TURN CLEAVES
C4 AND C2 TO FORM AN ENZYMATICALLY ACTIVE ASSOCIATION
COMPLEX DESIGNATED:
A.   C3 convertase
B.   C5
C.   Factor A of the properdin system
D.   Factor B of the properdin system
E.   C3 proactivator
Ref. Lepow, I. H. , Rosen, F. S. : Pathways to the Complement System.
New Eng J Med, 286:942, 1972.

968.   ALL OF THE FOLLOWING ARE HUMORAL FACTORS INVOLVED IN THE
INFLAMMATORY RESPONSE, EXCEPT:
A.   Histamine
B.   Serotonin
C.   Activated Hageman factor
D.   Dopamine
E.   Lysosomes
Ref. Hersh, E. M. , Bodey, G. P. : Leukocytic Mechanisms in
Inflammation. Ann Rev Med, 21:105, 1970.

969.   WHICH OF THE FOLLOWING IMMUNOLOGICAL FUNCTIONS ARE
ABNORMAL DURING STEROID TREATMENT?:
A.   In vitro lymphocyte transformation in response to candida antigens
B.   Agglutinating antibody response to candida antigens
C.   Quantitative indirect immunofluorescent antibodies using candida
antigens
D.   All of the above
Ref. Folb, P. I. , Trounce, J. R. : Immunological Aspects of Candida
Infection Complicating Steroid and Immunosuppressive Drug Therapy.
Lancet, 2:1112, 1970.

970.   THE SERUM IMMUNOGLOBULIN WHICH MAKES UP THE MAJORITY
OF HUMAN ANTIRABIES ANTIBODY 14 DAYS AFTER A COURSE OF
DUCK EMBRYO RABIES VACCINE IS:
A.   IgA   D.   IgD
B.   IgG   E.   IgE
C.   IgM
Ref. Rubin, R. H. , Gough, P. , Gerlach, E. H. : Immunoglobulin
Response to Rabies Vaccine in Man. Lancet, 1:625, 1971.

971.   THE CORRECT DOSE OF HUMAN TETANUS IMMUNE GLOBULIN FOR
PREVENTION OF TETANUS IS:
A.   30 units   D.   300 units
B.   3000 units   E.   80, 000 units
C.   1500 units
Ref. Prophylactic dose of Human Tetanus Immune Globulin. The
Medical Letter, 14:12, 1972.

972.   PLASMACYTES PRODUCING ANTIBODY IN THE PERIPHERAL
        LYMPHATIC TISSUES ARE DERIVED FROM:
        A. Thymus
        B. Bone marrow
        C. White pulp of the spleen
        D. Deep cortical areas of the lymph node
        E. Thoracic duct lymph
        Ref. Craddock, C. G. , Longmire, R. , McMillan, R. : Lymphocytes and
        the Immune Response. N Eng J Med, 285:378, 1971.

973.   THE MAJOR FACTOR CONTRIBUTING TO THE INCREASED INCIDENCE
        OF INFECTION OF THE LOWER EXTREMITIES IN DIABETIC
        PATIENTS IS:
        A. Increased nasal carriage of S. aureus
        B. Trauma due to neuropathy
        C. Peripheral vascular insufficiency
        D. Ketoacidosis
        E. Hyperglycemia
        Ref. Younger, D. : Infections and Diabetes. Med Clin N Amer, 49:1005,
        1965.

974.   DEFECTS IN WHICH OF THE FOLLOWING ARE NOTED IN PATIENTS
        WITH SEVERE INFECTIONS?:
        A. Phagocytosis   D. PMN migration
        B. Chemotaxis   E. All of the above
        C. Bactericidal activity
        Ref. Copeland, J. L. , Karrh, L. R. , McCoy, J. , Guckian, J. C. :
        Bactericidal Activity of Polymorphonuclear Leukocytes from Patients
        with Severe Bacterial Infections. Texas Rep Biol Med, 29:4, 1971.

975.   THE MOST CONSISTENT HEMOSTATIC DEFECT FOUND IN DISSEMINATED
        INTRAVASCULAR COAGULATION ASSOCIATED WITH INFECTION IS:
        A. Abnormally low plasma fibrinogen concentration
        B. Fibrin split products in excess of 6 micrograms/ml serum
        C. Depressed Factor V in plasma
        D. Thrombocytopenia
        E. Depressed Factor XII levels in plasma
        Ref. Yoshikawa, T. , Tanaka, K. R. , Guzel, B. : Infection and
        Disseminated Intravascular Coagulation. Medicine, 50:237, 1971.

976.   A SERIOUS LIMITATION ON APPLICATION OF THE LYMPHOCYTE
        TRANSFORMATION TECHNIQUE TO CLINICAL STUDIES IS:
        A. Prolonged period of time needed to obtain results
        B. Excessive bacterial contamination
        C. Large quantities of blood are needed
        D. Difficulty in obtaining purified lymphocyte suspension
        E. Excessive cost
        Ref. Parker, J. W. , Lukes, R. J. : A Microculture Method for Lymphocyte
        Transformation Studies in the Clinical Laboratory. Amer J Clin Path,
        56:174, 1971.

977.   ALL OF THE FOLLOWING ARE FUNCTIONS OF THE LYMPHATIC
        SYSTEM, EXCEPT:
        A. Provide antigenically determined specificity by opsonizing viable
            pathogenic particles
        B. Provide memory of previous antigenic experience
        C. Lysosomal enzyme activation
        D. Direct cytotoxicity
        Ref. Craddock, C. G. , Longmire, R. , McMillan, R. : Lymphocytes and
        the Immune Response. N Eng J Med, 285:324, 1971.

978. WHICH OF THE FOLLOWING IS THE MOST DESIRABLE PREPARATION
FOR BOOSTING DIPHTHERIA ANTITOXIN LEVELS IN AN ADULT WHO
HAS HAD NO IMMUNIZATION FOR 12 YEARS, BUT WAS PRIMARILY
IMMUNIZED IN CHILDHOOD?:
A. Diphtheria and tetanus toxoids and pertussis vaccine (DTP)
B. Tetanus toxoid
C. Tetanus and diphtheria toxoids, absorbed, adult type
D. Tetanus and diphtheria toxoids, fluid, adult type
E. Diphtheria toxoid
Ref. Diphtheria and Tetanus Toxoids and Pertussis Vaccine. Recom-
mendations of the Public Health Service Advisory Committee on
Immunization Practices. Ann Intern Med, 76:289, 1972.

979. WHICH OF THE FOLLOWING LEUKOCYTE FUNCTIONS ARE NORMAL
IN PATIENTS WITH CHRONIC GRANULOMATOUS DISEASE?:
A. O_2 consumption after phagocytosis
B. Lecithin synthesis during phagocytosis
C. NBT test
D. Iodination test
E. Glucose 1-C oxidation
Ref. Douglas, S.: Analytic Review: Disorders of Phagocyte Function.
Blood, 35:851, 1966.

980. A RENAL ALLOGRAFT (CARDAVERIC) PATIENT DEVELOPED A WIDE-
SPREAD INTERSTITIAL INFILTRATE INVOLVING MOST OF THE LEFT
LUNG. WHICH OF THE FOLLOWING EVENTS WOULD YOU ANTICIPATE
MOST LIKELY OCCURRED WITHIN 2 WEEKS OF THE APPEARANCE OF
PNEUMONIA?:
A. Rejection crisis
B. Reduction of prednisone dosage
C. Urinary tract infection
D. Reduction of 8-azothioprine dosage
E. None of the above
Ref. Briggs, W.A., Merrill, J.P., O'Brien, T.F., et al: Severe
Pneumonia in Transplant Patients. Ann Int Med, 75:887, 1971.

981. CELL-MEDIATED RESISTANCE IS THOUGHT TO BE OF PRIMARY
IMPORTANCE IN RESOLVING INFECTIONS CAUSED BY ALL OF THE
FOLLOWING ORGANISMS, EXCEPT:
A. M. tuberculosis
B. L. monocytogenes
C. S. typhosa
D. Streptococcus pyogenes
E. Brucella sp.
Ref. Mudd, S.: Resistance Against Staphylococcus Aureus. JAMA,
218:1671, 1971.

982. THE MOST COMMONLY IDENTIFIED ETIOLOGY FOR "FEVER OF
UNKNOWN ORIGIN" SYNDROME OCCURRING IN GENERAL HOSPITAL
POPULATIONS IS:
A. Neoplasm
B. Infection
C. Cirrhosis
D. Collagen disorders
E. Unknown
Ref. Deal, W.B.: Fever of Unknown Origin. Postgrad Med, 50:182, 1971.

983. THE OUTSTANDING FINDING AT AUTOPSY OF A SERIES OF PATIENTS
DYING FROM SEPTIC SHOCK WOULD BE:
A. Adrenal medullary necrosis
B. Acute renal tubular necrosis
C. Myocardial infarction
D. Widespread microthromboemboli
E. Unsuspected cholangitis
Ref. Neely, W. A., Berry, D. W., Rushton, F. W., et al: Septic Shock.
Ann Surg, 173:657, 1971.

984. THE MOST COMMON COEXISTING DISEASE ACCOMPANYING PRO-
LONGED SALMONELLA BACTEREMIA ("PROLONGED TYPHOID
FEVER") IS:
A. Diabetes mellitus
B. Biliary tract disease
C. Schistosomiasis
D. Hemoglobinopathy
E. Addison's disease
Ref. Rocha, H., Kirk, J. W., Hearey, D. C., Jr.: Prolonged Salmonella
Bacteremia in Patients with Schistosoma Mansoni Infection. Arch Int Med,
128:254, 1971.

THE FOLLOWING QUESTIONS CONSIST OF PAIRS OF PHRASES
DESCRIBING CONDITIONS OR QUANTITIES WHICH MAY OR MAY NOT
VARY IN RELATION TO EACH OTHER. ANSWER:
A. If increase in the first is accompanied by increase in the second or
decrease in the first is accompanied by decrease in the second
B. If increase in the first is accompanied by decrease in the second or
decrease in the first is accompanied by increase in the second
C. If changes in the first are independent of changes in the second

985. 1. Phagocytosis of S. aureus by normal human neutrophilic leukocytes
in vitro
2. Glucose concentration of medium in which normal leukocytes are
suspended (lower limit of 50mg %)
Ref. Van Oss, C. J.: Influence of Glucose Levels on the In Vitro
Phagocytosis of Bacteria by Human Neutrophils. Inf and Imm, 4:54, 1971.

THE FOLLOWING QUESTIONS CONSIST OF A STATEMENT AND A
REASON. SELECT:
A. If both statement and reason are true and the reason is a correct
explanation of the statement
B. If both statement and reason are true but the reason is not a correct
explanation of the statement
C. If the statement is true but the reason is false
D. If the statement is false but the reason is true
E. If both statement and reason are false

986. ____ Multiple injections of endotoxin increase the resistance of experimental
animals to lethal shock BECAUSE acquired resistance produced by
multiple injections of endotoxin is specific for the endotoxin used to
immunize an experimental animal.
Ref. Gram Negative Sepsis, Sanford, J. P., (Ed), Med Com, New York,
N. Y., 1971, p. 38.

987. ___ Blood and urine cultures should be obtained from all newborn babies with jaundice BECAUSE jaundice caused by infection may be present even though the newborn infant does not appear to be ill.
Ref. Rooney, J. C. , Hill, D. J. , Danks, D. M. : Jaundice Associated with Bacterial Infection in the Newborn. Amer J Dis Child, 122:39, 1971.

988. ___ Management of bacteruria in boys requires urologic investigation BECAUSE bacteruria in boys is almost invariably accompanied by urinary tract obstruction or anatomic abnormality.
Ref. Kunin, C. M. , Pacquin, J. A. : Frequency and Natural History of Urinary Tract Infections in School Children in Progress in Pyelonephritis. Kass, E. H. , (Ed), Philadelphia, Davis, 1965, p. 33.

989. ___ Immunization of man with antigens from one strain of Pseudomonas may not protect man from invasion by Pseudomonas BECAUSE immunity following Pseudomonas infections is mainly type-specific.
Ref. Crowder, J. G. , Fisher, M. W. , White, A. : Type-Specific Immunity in Pseudomonas Disease. J Lab Clin Med. 79:47, 1972.

990. ___ Serum bactericidal antibody may be a critical determinant of host resistance to infection by Hemophilus influenzae, type B, BECAUSE H. influenzae B infections of agammaglobulinemic children are largely prevented by administration of gamma globulin.
Ref. Anderson, P. , Johnson, R. B. , Jr. , Smith, D. H. : Human Serum Activities Against Hemophilus Influenzae, Type B. J Clin Invest, 51:31, 1972.

991. ___ Cholera skin toxin produces a firm, erythematous swelling when injected intracutaneously into the skin of non-immune humans BECAUSE the cholera skin toxin is absorbed from the gut and elicits an antibody response.
Ref. Craig, J. P. , Eichner, E. , Hornick, R. B. : Cutaneous Responses to Cholera Skin Toxin in Man; L Responses in Unimmunized American Males. J Infect Dis, 125:203, 1972.

992. ___ Patients with gram negative bacteremia who have evidence of low cardiac output and vasoconstriction should be treated vigorously for concomitant hypovolemia or cardiac disease BECAUSE the species of gram negative bacteria causing sepsis has little effect on the hemodynamic changes.
Ref. Wilson, R. F. , Sawer, E. J. , LeBlanco, P. L. : Factors Affecting Hemodynamics in Clinical Shock with Sepsis. Ann Surg, 174:939, 1971.

993. ___ Human mononuclear cells are a major source of endogenous pyrogen BECAUSE blood cells from patients with agranulocytosis release large amounts of endogenous pyrogen when these cells are incubated with heat-killed staphylococci.
Ref. Atkins, E. , Bodel, P. : Fever. New Eng J Med, 286:27, 1972.

994. ___ Disseminated intravascular coagulation produced by infection leads to hypocoagulable blood BECAUSE of inhibition of fibrin polymerization by fibrin split products.
Ref. Yoshikawa, T. , Tanaka, K. R. , Guze, L. B. : Infection and Disseminated Intravascular Coagulation. Medicine, 50:237, 1971.

995.   Detection of pyuria in a clean-catch urine sample is not a reliable
___   indication of bacteruria BECAUSE leukocyte excretion in the urine is
        appreciably influenced by changes in urine volume, osmolality, and
        techniques of examination.
        Ref. Lang, G. R. , Levin, S.: Diagnosis and Treatment of Urinary
        Tract Infections. Med Clin N Amer, 55:1439, 1971.

996.   Skin testing with penicilloyl-polylysine and minor determinant mixture
___   will identify patients whose history includes penicillin allergy but
        who can safely receive penicillin BECAUSE negative reactions to both
        penicilloyl-polylysine and minor determinant mixture are not associated
        with immediate or anaphylactic reactions to penicillin.
        Ref. Levine, B. B.: Skin Rashes with Penicillin Therapy: Current
        Management. New Eng J Med, 286:42, 1972.

997.   Neonatal thymectomy facilitates development of immune paralysis
___   BECAUSE the capacity to produce a secondary antibody response is
        depressed much more following thymectomy than is the capacity to
        produce a primary antibody response.
        Ref. Lemmel, E-M, Cooper, M. D. , Good, R. A.: Neonatal Thymectomy
        and the Antibody Response to Sheep Erythrocytes in Mice. Int Arch All
        Appl Immunol, 41:873, 1971.

998.   Transfusion of fresh blood or plasma is therapeutically useful for
___   children with phagocytic defects BECAUSE the specific deficiency of
        impaired phagocytosis is abnormal C5 which can be corrected by
        transfusion of fresh blood or plasma.
        Ref. Miller, M. E.: Enhanced Susceptibility to Infection. Med Clin N
        Amer, 54:713, 1970.

        ANSWER THE FOLLOWING QUESTIONS ACCORDING TO THE KEY
        BELOW:
        A. If choice A is greater then choice B
        B. If choice B is greater than choice A
        C. If A and B are equal or nearly equal

999.   THE PRODUCTION OF HEMAGGLUTINATING OR BACTERICIDAL
        ANTIBODIES BY CHILDREN WITH HEMOPHILUS INFLUENZAE
        MENINGITIS WHO ARE:
        A. Less than 2 years old
        B. More than 2 years old
        Ref. Norden, C. W. , Melish, M. , Overall, J. A. , et al: Immunologic
        Responses to Hemophilus Influenzae Meningitis. J Ped, 80:209, 1972.

1000.   SERUM HALF LIFE $(T\frac{1}{2})$ OF:
        A. Rabies immune globulin of human origin
        B. Homologous immune globulin
        Ref. Cabasso, V. J. , Loofbourow, J. C. , Roby, R. E. , Anuskiewicz, W.:
        Rabies Immune Globulin of Human Origin: Preparation and Dosage
        Determinations in Non-Exposed Volunteer Subjects. Bull Wld Hlth Org,
        45:303, 1971.

1001.   POSTPHAGOCYTIC INCREASE IN OXYGEN CONSUMPTION AND
        HYDROGEN PEROXIDE PRODUCTION BY LEUKOCYTES INGESTING:
        A. Polystyrene latex spheres (1.08 microns)
        B. Heat killed staphylococcus (0.8 microns)
        Ref. Mandell, G. L.: Influence of Type of Ingested Particle on Human
        Leukocyte Metabolism. Prox Soc Exp Biol Med, 137:1228, 1971.

1002.   JOINT FLUID/SERUM COMPLEMENT RATIO IN JOINT EFFUSION
        FLUID ASSOCIATED WITH:
        A. Systemic lupus erythematosus
        B. Infections of the joint
        Ref. Cracchiola, A.: Joint Fluid Analysis. Family Physician, 87,
        November 1971.

1003.   RESPONSE OF PATIENT WITH NEUTROPHIL COUNT OF:
        A. 50/cu mm to treatment with gentamicin for infection caused by
            gentamicin-sensitive bacteria
        B. 1250/cu mm to treatment with gentamicin under similar circumstance
        Ref. Bodey, G. P., Middleman, E., Umswasadi, T., et al: Intravenous
        Gentamicin Therapy for Infections in Patients with Cancer. J Inf Dis,
        124(S):174, 1971.

1004.   AMOUNT OF C3 IN SERUM OF:
        A. Normal persons
        B. Patients with defective leukocyte phagocytosis
        Ref. Miller, M. E., Enhanced Susceptibility to Infection. Med Clin
        N Amer, 54:713, 1970.

1005.   THE NUMBER OF PATIENTS WITH AUTHENTICATED HISTORIES OF
        IMMEDIATE HYPERSENSITIVITY TO PENICILLIN WHO WILL HAVE
        A POSITIVE INTRADERMAL TEST USING:
        A. Penicillin G
        B. Penicilloyl-polylysine
        Ref. Green, G. R., Rosenblum, A.: Report of the Penicillin Study
        Group - American Academy of Allergy. J All Clin Immunol, 48:331,
        1971.

        EACH SET OF LETTERED HEADINGS IS FOLLOWED BY A NUMBERED
        LIST OF WORDS OR PHRASES. ANSWER:
        A. If the word or phrase is associated with A only
        B. If the word or phrase is associated with B only
        C. If the word or phrase is associated with A and B
        D. If the word or phrase is associated with neither A nor B

        A. Macrophage aggregation factor
        B. Migration inhibition factor
        C. Both
        D. Neither

1006.   ___ Assay utilizes non-sensitive cell population
1007.   ___ Reflects delayed hypersensitivity
1008.   ___ Produced by incubation of sensitive lymphocyte with specific antigen
1009.   ___ Independent of humoral antibody
        Ref. Gotoff, S. P., Vizral, I. F.: The Macrophage Aggregation Assay
        for Delayed Hypersensitivity: Development of the Response, Role of the
        Macrophage, and the Independence of Humoral Antibody. Cell Immunol,
        3:53, 1972.

A. Alum-precipitated toxoid
B. Live vaccine
C. Both
D. Neither

010. ___ Diphtheria
011. ___ Diphtheria-tetanus-pertussis-poliomyelitis
012. ___ Influenza
013. ___ Smallpox
014. ___ Tetanus
015. ___ BCG
016. ___ Rabies
017. ___ Measles
Ref. Fekety, F. R. , Allen, J. C. , Cluff, L. E. : Management of Infectious Diseases in The Principles and Practice of Medicine, 17th Ed, Chap 67, Appleton-Century-Crofts, New York, 1968, pp. 671-686.

A. Thymus-dependent lymphocytes
B. Bursa-dependent lymphocytes
C. Both
D. Neither

1018. ___ Bone marrow origin
1019. ___ Days-to-weeks life span
1020. ___ Majority of recirculating lymphocyte pool
1021. ___ Antibody synthesis
1022. ___ Cell-mediated immunity
1023. ___ Phytohemagglutinin response
1024. ___ Germinal centers of lymph nodes
1025. ___ Antigen processing
Ref. Craddock, C. G. , Longmire, R. , McMillan, R. : Lymphocytes and the Immune Response. N Eng J Med, 285:324, 1971.

IN THE FOLLOWING QUESTIONS, CHOOSE:
A. If 1, 2 and 3 are correct
B. If 1 and 3 are correct
C. If 2 and 4 are correct
D. If only 4 is correct
E. If all 4 are correct

1026. FECAL POLYMORPHONUCLEAR LEUKOCYTES ARE CHARACTERISTI-CALLY SEEN IN THE STOOL OF PATIENTS WITH:
1. Shigellosis
2. Experimentally-induced typhoid fever
3. Salmonellosis
4. Viral gastroenteritis
Ref. Harris, J. C. , DuPont, H. , Hornic, R. B. : Fecal Leukocytes in Diarrheal Illness. Ann Intern Med, 76:697, 1972.

1027. EXTRACTS OR PRODUCTS OF THE FOLLOWING MICROORGANISMS HAVE BEEN SHOWN TO HAVE IMMUNOSUPRESSIVE ACTIVITY:
1. P. aeruginosa
2. B. pertussis
3. S. typhi
4. S. paratyphi B
Ref. Floersheim, G. L. , Hopff, W. H. , Gasser, M. , et al: Impairment of Cell Mediated Immune Response by Pseudomonas Aeruginosa.
Clin Exp Immunol, 9:241, 1971.

1028.   WHICH OF THE FOLLOWING FACTORS TEND TO REDUCE THE
        INTENSITY AND SEVERITY OF RESPIRATORY TRACT INFECTIONS A:
        A CHILD GROWS OLDER?:
        1. Frequent infections in early life
        2. Infrequent exposure in the home
        3. Born before 1946
        4. Tonsillectomy and adenoidectomy
        Ref. McCammon, R. W.: Natural History of Respiratory Tract Infection
        Patterns in Basically Healthy Individuals. JAMA, 122:232, 1971.

1029.   WHICH OF THE FOLLOWING STATEMENTS CONCERNING
        PNEUMOCOCCAL BACTEREMIA AND MENINGITIS IN PATIENTS WITH
        SICKLE CELL ANEMIA IS (ARE) CORRECT?:
        1. About 85% of such patients are less than 3 years old
        2. A small number of pneumococcal types are responsible
        3. Patients are usually functionally asplenic
        4. Pneumococcal serum opsonins are present in normal amounts
        Ref. Lukens, J. N.: Hemoglobin S, the Pneumococcus, and the Spleen.
        Amer J Dis Child, 123:6, 1972.

1030.   THE PREDOMINANT TYPE OF CELL EXCRETED IN THE SPUTUM IN
        CHRONIC BRONCHIAL INFLAMMATION OF NON-ALLERGIC NATURE
        IS (ARE):
        1. Neutrophils
        2. Histiocytes
        3. Bronchial epithelial cells
        4. Plasma cells
        Ref. Medici, T. C., Chodosh, S.: Sputum Cell Dynamics in Bacterial
        Exacerbations of Chronic Bronchial Disease. Arch Intern Med,
        129:597, 1972.

1031.   THE SITES OF FATAL INFECTION IN CHILDHOOD LEUKEMIA ARE
        USUALLY:
        1. Sepsis
        2. Pneumonia
        3. Entercolitis
        4. Pyoderma
        Ref. Hughes, W. T.: Fatal Infections in Childhood Leukemia.
        Am J Dis Child, 122:283, 1971.

1032.   ABNORMAL OR DEFECTIVE POLYMORPHONUCLEAR LEUKOCYTE
        CHEMOTAXIS HAS BEEN DEMONSTRATED IN:
        1. Cirrhotic patients
        2. Chediak-Higashi syndrome
        3. SLE
        4. Diabetes mellitus
        Ref. DeMeo, A., Andersen, B. R.: Defective Chemotaxis Associated
        with a Serum Inhibitor in Cirrhotic Patients. New Eng J Med,
        286:735, 1972.

1033.   THE REASONS FOR FULMINANT PNEUMOCOCCAL INFECTIONS IN
        CHILDREN WITH SICKLE CELL ANEMIA ARE:
        1. Leukopenia
        2. Functional asplenia
        3. Hypothermia
        4. Deficient serum opsonins for pneumococci
        Ref. Seeler, R. A., Metzer, W., Mufson, M. A.: Diplococcus Pneumoniae
        Infections in Children with Sickle Cell Anemia. Amer J Dis Child,
        123:8, 1972.

034.   HEPARIN SHOULD BE USED WITH GREAT CAUTION IN THE TREAT-
       MENT OF CONSUMPTION COAGULOPATHY IF:
       1. Fibrin split products are circulating in the serum in large quantities
       2. There is uncorrected hypofibrinogenemia (less than 50 mg/100ml)
       3. There is associated inflammatory vasculitis
       4. There is thrombocytopenia
       Ref. Green, D. , Seeler, R. A. , Allen, N. , et al: The Role of Heparin
       in the Management of Consumption Coagulopathy. Med Clin N Amer,
       56:193, 1972.

1035.   THE FACTORS RESPONSIBLE FOR THE LETHAL ACTION OF NORMAL
        HUMAN SERUM ON L-PHASE VARIANTS OF BACTERIA ARE:
        1. Lysosome
        2. Serum complement
        2. Beta-lysin
        4. Serum antibody
        Ref. McGee, Z. A. , Ratner, H. B. , Bryant, R. E. , et al: An Antibody
        Complement System in Human Serum Lethal to L-Phase Variants of
        Bacteria. J Infect Dis, 125:231, 1972.

1036.   PATIENTS WITH CHEDIAK-HIGASHI SYNDROME DEMONSTRATE
        WHICH OF THE FOLLOWING ABNORMALITIES IN LEUKOCYTE
        FUNCTION?:
        1. Neutropenia
        2. Defective leukocyte migration
        3. Failure of post phagocytic degranulation
        4. Reduced quantities of lysosomal enzymes
        Ref. Wolff, S. , Dale, D. C. , Clark, R. A. , et al: The Chediak-Higashi
        Syndrome: Studies of Host Defenses. Ann Intern Med, 76:293, 1972.

1037.   INTRALEUKOCYTIC MICROBICIDAL SYSTEMS INCLUDE:
        1. Fall in pH
        2. H_2O_2 production
        3. Myeloperoxidase
        4. IgM antibodies
        Ref. Klebanoff, S. J. : Intraleukocytic Microbicidal Defects. Ann Rev
        Med, 22:39, 1971.

1038.   THE METABOLIC "BURST" OF LEUKOCYTES DURING PHAGOCYTOSIS
        INCLUDES:
        1. Increased O_2 consumption
        2. Increased H_2O_2 production
        3. Increased activity of the hexosemonophosphate shunt
        4. Decreased lecithin synthesis
        Ref. Miller, M. E. : Enhanced Susceptibility to Infection. Med Clin N
        Amer, 54:713, 1970.

1039.   WHICH OF THE FOLLOWING LEUKOCYTIC PROPERTIES ARE
        DEPRESSED IN THE CHEDIAK-HIGASHI SYNDROME?:
        1. Phagocytosis
        2. Phagosomal acid phosphatase content
        3. Phagosomal alkaline phosphatase content
        4. Phagosomal peroxidase content
        Ref. Stossel, T. P. , Root, R. K. , Vaughan, M. : Phagocytosis in
        Chronic Granulomatous Disease and the Chediak-Higashi Syndrome.
        New Eng J Med, 286:120, 1972.

1040.   COMPARING "TOXIC" NEUTROPHILES APPEARING DURING THE
         COURSE OF SEVERE INFECTION TO NEUTROPHILES OBTAINED FROM
         NORMAL PERSONS, THE FOLLOWING CHANGES ARE FOUND:
         1.   Cytoplasmic vacuoles appear in toxic neutrophiles
         2.   Lysosomal alkaline phosphatase increases in toxic neutrophiles
         3.   Chemotactic activity of toxic neutrophiles is decreased compared to
              controls
         4.   Toxic neutrophiles migrate more slowly from glass tubes than do
              normal neutrophiles
         Ref. McCall, C. E., Caves, J., Cooper, R., DeChatelet, L.: Functional
         Characteristics of Human Toxic Neutrophils. J Infect Dis, 124:68, 1971.

1041.   INFECTIOUS DISEASES IN WHICH IMMUNE COMPLEXES HAVE BEEN
         IMPLICATED IN AN ASSOCIATED NEPHROPATHY INCLUDE:
         1.   Infected ventriculo-atrial shunts
         2.   Syphilis
         3.   Osteomyelitis
         4.   Infectious mononucleosis
         Ref. Gutman, R. A., Striker, G. A., Gilliland, B. C., et al: The Immune
         Complex Glomerulonephritis of Bacterial Endocarditis. Medicine, 51:1,
         1972.

1042.   THE FOLLOWING ARE CHARACTERISTICS OF CHRONIC GRANULO-
         MATOUS DISEASE:
         1.   Normal leukocytic lysosomal contents
         2.   Normal increase in lecithin synthesis during phagocytosis
         3.   Deficient intracellular generation of H_2O_2 by leukocyte
         4.   Normal phagocytosis of bacteria
         Ref. Miller, M. E.: Enhanced Susceptibility to Infection. Med Clin N
         Amer, 54:722, 1970.

1043.   WHICH OF THE FOLLOWING MATERNAL EVENTS IS CLEARLY
         RELATED TO CONGENITAL PNEUMONIA OF THE NEWBORN?:
         1.   Chorioamnionitis
         2.   Multiparity
         3.   Urinary tract infection (antenatal)
         4.   Obesity
         Ref. Naeye, R. L., Dellinger, W. S., Blanc, W. A.: Fetal and Maternal
         Features of Antenatal Bacterial Infections. J Pediatrics, 79:733, 1971.

1044.   THE RESPONSE OF MAN TO INDUCED INFECTION WITH SALMONELLA
         TYPHOSA, PASTURELLA TULARENSIS, SANDFLY FEVER VIRUS, AND
         PRESUMABLY A NUMBER OF OTHER MICROORGANISMS INCLUDES:
         1.   Initial decrease in serum amino acids
         2.   Increase in serum haptoglobin
         3.   Increase in serum glycoprotein
         4.   No initial change in excretion of amino acids
         Ref. Wannemacher, R. W., Powanda, M. C., Pekarek, R. S., et al:
         Tissue Amino Acid Flux After Exposure of Rats to Diplococcus
         Pneumoniae. Infect and Imm, 4:556, 1971.

1045.   A POSITIVE NITROBLUE TETRAZOLIUM REDUCTION TEST (MORE
        THAN 11% OF NEUTROPHILES CONTAINING FORMOZAN DEPOSITS)
        IS FOUND IN:
        1. Malaria
        2. Chronic mucocutaneous candidiasis
        3. Active pyogenic infections
        4. Pneumocystis carinii pneumonia
        Ref. Matula, G., Paterson, P.Y.: Spontaneous in Vitro Reduction of
        Nitroblue Tetrazolium by Neutrophils of Adult Patients with Bacterial
        Infection. N Eng J Med, 285:311, 1971.

1046.   THE CONTRIBUTION OF THE LYMPHATIC SYSTEM TO BODY DEFENSE
        INCLUDES:
        1. Opsonizing pathogenic particles for phagocytosis
        2. Develop lymphoid cells that directly damage the pathogen
        3. Memory of previous experience
        4. Lysosomal enzyme activation
        Ref. Craddock, C.G., Longmire, R., McMillan, R.: Lymphocytes
        and the Immune Response. NEJ Med, 285:324, 1971.

1047.   THE NITROBLUE TETRAZOLIUM REDUCTION TEST BY
        NEUTROPHILES WOULD BE EXPECTED TO BE POSITIVE IN THE
        FOLLOWING SITUATIONS:
        1. Untreated E. coli bacteremia
        2. Active pulmonary tuberculosis
        3. Actue suppurative appendicitis
        4. Disseminated carcinomatosis
        Ref. Matula, G., Paterson, P.Y.: Spontaneous in Vitro Reduction of
        Nitroblue Tetrazolium by Neutrophils of Adult Patients with Bacterial
        Infection. New Eng J Med, 285:311, 1971.

1048.   THE FOLLOWING PATHOLOGIC STATES MAY BE RESPONSIBLE FOR
        THE INITIATION OF DISSEMINATED INTRAVASCULAR COAGULATION:
        1. Clostridium perfringens bacteremia
        2. Staphylococcal sepsis
        3. Rubella
        4. Rocky Mountain spotted fever
        Ref. Yoshikawa, T., Tanaka, K.R., Guze, L.: Infection and
        Disseminated Intravascular Coagulation. Medicine, 50:237, 1971.

1049.   THE FOLLOWING ARE CHARACTERISTICS OF CHRONIC GRANULO-
        MATOUS DISEASE:
        1. Humoral immune responses are normal
        2. Typically found in females
        3. Defective bactericidal capacity of polymorphonuclear leukocytes
        4. Cellular immune responses are deficient
        Ref. Balfour, H.H., Shehan, J.J., Speicher, C.E., Kauder, E.:
        Chronic Granulomatous Disease of Childhood in a 23 Year-Old Man.
        JAMA, 217:960, 1971.

EACH GROUP OF ITEMS CONSISTS OF A LIST OF LETTERED
HEADINGS FOLLOWED BY A LIST OF NUMBERED WORDS OR
PHRASES. FOR EACH NUMBERED WORD OR PHRASE, SELECT THE
ONE HEADING MOST CLOSELY RELATED TO IT:

A. Anemia nearly universal with infection
B. Anemia sporadically present with infection - probably on an
    immune basis
C. Causal association of anemia with infection is speculative

1050. ___ Mycoplasma pneumonia
1051. ___ Malaria
1052. ___ Clostridial sepsis
1053. ___ Miliary tuberculosis
1054. ___ Hookworm disease
1055. ___ Oroya fever
    Ref. Barrett-Conner, E.: Anemia and Infection. Amer J Med,
    52:242, 1972.

PROCOAGULANTS MAY ENTER THE CIRCULATION AND INITIATE
DISSEMINATED INTRAVASCULAR COAGULATION. MATCH THE
PROCOAGULANT WITH THE APPROPRIATE DISEASE AS A SOURCE
OF THE PROCOAGULANT:

A. Bacterial endotoxin
B. Procoagulants from erythrocytes
C. Damage to endothelial cells
D. Tissue thromboplastins

1056. ___ Malaria
1057. ___ Gram negative septicemia
1058. ___ Rocky Mountain spotted fever
1059. ___ Carcinomatosis
    Ref. Kwaan, H.C.: Disseminated Intravascular Coagulation.
    Med Clin N Amer, 56:177, 1972.

A. Anaphylatoxin
B. Factor XII
C. Prostaglandins
D. Serotonin
E. Opsonins

1060. ___ Amine originating mainly from mast cells
1061. ___ Cleavage product of C5
1062. ___ Activation of kinin System
1063. ___ Long chain lipids
1064. ___ Antibodies fixed on surface of particle to be phagocytosed
    Ref. Movat, H.Z.: The Acute Inflammatory Reaction in Inflammation,
    Immunity, and Hypersensitivity. Harper and Row, New York, 1971,
    pp. 1-130.

A. IgG
B. IgA
C. IgM
D. IgD
E. IgE

1065. ___ Reagenic antibody; elevated in patients with allergic manifestations
1066. ___ Intravascular location; usually first immunoglobulin to appear
      following immunization
1067. ___ No known function
1068. ___ Serum and secretory forms
1069. ___ Predominant immunoglobulin in extracellular fluids
      Ref. Waldman, R. H. : Immune Mechanisms on Secretory Surfaces.
      Postgrad Med, 50:78, 1971.

STUDY THE CASE HISTORY AND SELECT THE MOST APPROPRIATE
ANSWER TO EACH QUESTION:

CASE HISTORY (QUESTIONS 1070-1073)
In January, a 22 year-old high school teacher developed fever, chills,
headache, and extra-ocular myalgia within an 8-hour period. A similar
syndrome was commonly seen in her school and the community at that
time. For 12 years she had been followed by her personal physician
because of rheumatic heart disease with minimal mitral stenosis.
Within 24 hours she sought medical attention because of shortness of
breath. On examination she was agitated, sitting erect, and manifested
peri-oral cyanosis. T - 40°C; R - 48/min; BP 100/70; P - 120/min

1070. PHYSICAL EXAMINATION OF THE CHEST WOULD MOST LIKELY
       REVEAL:
       A. Flat percussion note at the right base
       B. Absent breath sounds over one entire hemithorax
       C. Diffuse moist rales
       D. Post-effort breathing
       E. Marked bronchial breathing

1071. THE CHEST X-RAY WILL PROBABLY REVEAL:
       A. Pneumothorax
       B. Diffuse bilateral nodular infiltrates
       C. Lobar pneumonia
       D. Pleural effusion
       E. Normal findings

1072. BLOOD CULTURES WOULD BE EXPECTED TO REVEAL:
       A. Hemophilus influenzae
       B. Staphylococcus aureus
       C. Diplococcus pneumoniae
       D. No organisms
       E. None of the above

1073. THE THERAPEUTIC APPROACH MOST LIKELY TO PREVENT DEATH
       UNDER THESE CIRCUMSTANCES IS:
       A. Amantadine hydrochloride
       B. Bronchodilators
       C. Steroid therapy
       D. Appropriate antibiotics
       E. None of the above
       Ref. Kilbourne, E. D.: Influenza in Textbook of Medicine, Ed by Beeson,
       P. B., McDermott, W., W. B. Saunders Co., Philadelphia, 1971, p. 368.

CASE HISTORY (QUESTION 1074)
A 71 year-old man had recently been discharged from a hospital
where the diagnosis of adenocarcinoma of the colon had been established.
One week later he was readmitted for complaints of fever of 2 days
duration. On admission he was acutely ill. The temperature was
38.5°C rectally. Blood pressure was 60/o. He received treatment
with vasopressors, ampicillin, and intravenous fluid replacement and
recovered rapidly. Four blood cultures obtained prior to treatment
all contained Cl. tertium.

1074. THE LEAST LIKELY ASSOCIATED FINDING WOULD BE:
A. Leukocytosis
B. Gas gangrene of the colon
C. Congestive heart failure
D. Bowel obstruction
E. Peritonitis
Ref. Alpern, R. J., Dowell, V. R., Jr.: Nonhistotoxic Clostridial
Bacteremia. Am J Clin Path, 55:717, 1971.

CASE HISTORY (QUESTION 1075)
A 37 year-old man underwent surgery for removal of a colloid cyst
from the third ventricle. Postoperatively he received tetracycline,
oxacillin, and erythromycin. Twenty-five days after surgery he
became febrile. Fever persisted despite treatment with penicillin
and chloramphenicol. A lumbar puncture revealed that the cerebrospinal fluid contained 4000 leukocytes/cu. mm., 75% of which were
polymorphonuclear leukocytes. A culture of the cerebrospinal fluid
contained a very mucoid gram-negative bacillus growing on blood and
EMB agar. The bacteriologist suspected that the organism was a
mucoid variant of P. aeruginosa.

1075. WHICH OF THE FOLLOWING WOULD PROVIDE A POSITIVE
IDENTIFICATION OF PSEUDOMONAS SPECIES?:
A. Citrate utilization
B. Pigment formation
C. Absence of hydrogen sulfide production
D. Sensitivity to gentamicin
E. Fermentation of glucose
Ref. Dalton, A.C., Smith, G. M.: Mucoid Pseudomonas Aeruginosa
Causing Meningitis. Am J Clin Path, 55:723, 1971.

CASE HISTORY (QUESTIONS 1076-1078)
A 68 year-old man, previously in good health, suddenly developed
sore throat, myalgia, headache, nonproductive cough, and mild
conjunctivitis. Epidemic influenza was occurring in the community
at the same time. Five days later he became restless, cyanotic and
tachypneic. Chest X-ray showed extensive bilateral lower lobe
pneumonia.

1076. WHAT IS THE MOST LIKELY PATHOLOGIC PROCESS IN THE LUNGS?:
A. Necrotizing hemorrhagic pneumonia
B. Diffuse alveolar cell wall thickening
C. Extensive early cavitation
D. Multiple pulmonary emboli
E. Diffuse bronchial hyperplasia

1077.   THE PATHOGEN MOST OFTEN RECOVERED FROM THE LUNG IN
         THIS CLINICAL SETTING IS:
         A. S. aureus   D. Influenza virus
         B. D. pneumoniae   E. None of the above
         C. P. aeruginosa

1078.   IF SUSPECTED, WHICH OF THE FOLLOWING WOULD BE THE
         QUICKEST MEANS OF IDENTIFYING INFLUENZA VIRUS INFECTION?:
         A. Paired sera for complement fixing antibody titer against influenza
             virus
         B. Blood culture
         C. Throat culture
         D. Stool culture
         E. Cytologic examination of the sputum
         Ref. Lindsay, M. E. , Morrow, G. W. : Primary Influenzal Pneumonia.
         Postgrad Med, 49:173, 1971.

         CASE HISTORY (QUESTIONS 1079-1080)
         A 56 year-old man awoke with headache, difficulty in speaking and
         swallowing, and weakness along the left side of the body. A tooth had
         been removed 10 days earlier without incident. On examination he
         had paralysis of cranial nerves V, VII, and VIII on the left plus a
         left hemiparesis. There was low grade fever. The spinal fluid was
         unremarkable. The next day he became semicomatose and died
         2 hours later. At autopsy an abscess in the right fronto-parietal
         area of the brain was identified,from which Hemophilus aphrophilus
         was cultured.

1079.   ANTIBIOTICS KNOWN TO BE EFFECTIVE AGAINST THIS ORGANISM
         INCLUDE:
         A. Ampicillin   D. Cephalosporin
         B. Penicillin   E. All of the above
         C. Streptomycin

1080.   EPIDEMIOLOGICAL INVESTIGATION MIGHT REVEAL:
         A. Close contact with birds
         B. Recent exposure to a patient with pneumonia
         C. Close contact with dogs
         D. Recent spelunking expedition
         E. None of the above
         Ref. Clapper, W. E. , Smith, E. A. : Hemophilus Aphrophilus in
         Brain Abscess. Amer J Clin Path, 55:726, 1971.

CASE HISTORY (QUESTIONS 1081-1082)

In August, an 18 year-old camper returned from a trip through a remote brushy area. During the trip he acquired numerous insect bites. Five days later he developed a frontal headache, mild chill, and fever of 101°F. On the first day of the illness he developed bone pain, photophobia, and arthralgia. On the second day there was fever of 104°F, and a macular measles-like rash developed. On the third day there was a petachial element to the eruption. The hematocrit, hemoglobin, WBC count, differential count, urinalysis, and platelet count were within the normal range.

1081. WHICH OF THE FOLLOWING WOULD APPLY ON THE FOURTH DAY OF ILLNESS?:
A. Proteus OX-19 agglutination reactions will be positive
B. Only Proteus OX-2 agglutination reactions will be positive
C. Both Proteus OX-19 and OX-2 agglutination reactions will be positive
D. Proteus agglutination reactions will be negative; complement fixation reactions with yolk sac antigen will be positive
E. None of the above

1082. PREFERRED TREATMENT INCLUDES THE USE OF:
A. Para-amino benzoic acid
B. Chloramphenicol
C. Tetracycline
D. Ampicillin
E. Sulfonamides

Ref. Ley, H.: Rocky Mountain Spotted Fever in Textbook of Medicine, Ed, Beeson, P. B., McDermott, W., 1971, W. B. Saunders Co., Philadelphia, p. 478.

CASE HISTORY (QUESTIONS 1083-1084)

A 25 year-old man developed stiffness, pain, swelling and heat in the joints of the hands, wrists, knees, hips, and spine. He used heroin intravenously. There was fusiform swelling of the proximal interphalangeal joints of both hands. Effusions were present in both knees. No rash was present. After 5 days of aspirin therapy he became jaundiced. At the same time all signs of arthritis disappeared. Liver function tests showed elevated bilirubin, SGOT, and normal alkaline phosphatase levels.

1083. THE MOST LIKELY CAUSE OF THE ARTHRITIS WAS:
A. Gonococcal arthritis   D. Syphilis
B. Lupus erythematosus   E. Rheumatoid arthritis
C. Infectious hepatitis

1084. WHICH OF THE FOLLOWING TESTS WOULD BE DIAGNOSTIC?:
A. Rheumatoid factor determination
B. Australia antigen determination in joint fluid
C. Antistreptolysin O serum titer
D. Lupus erythematosus cell preparation
E. Serum uric acid determination

Ref. Onion, D. K., Crumpacker, C. S., Gilliland, B. G.: Arthritis of Hepatitis Associated with Australia Antigen. Ann Intern Med, 75:29, 1971.

CASE HISTORY (QUESTIONS 1085-1087)
A 27 year-old diabetic presented with a 2 day history of vomiting,
fever, left frontal pain and swelling of the left eye. She became
lethargic and presented in semicoma. Examination revealed proptosis
of the left eye, blindness, and ophthalmoplegia of the left eye.
Laboratory studies showed diabetic ketoacidosis.

1085.   WHICH OF THE FOLLOWING ASSOCIATED FINDINGS WOULD BE MOST
ANTICIPATED?:
A. Extensive pyorrhea
B. Normal spinal fluid examination
C. Lung abscess
D. Dental abscess
E. Cloudiness of maxillary sinus

1086.   IF PHYCOMYCOSIS WAS PRESENT, BIOPSIES OR INFECTED
SECRETIONS WOULD CONTAIN:
A. Branching nonseptate hyphae
B. Budding yeast forms with a wide base
C. Branching septate hyphae
D. Acid-fast hyphae
E. Round, double-walled structures

1087.   WHICH OF THE FOLLOWING IS A MAJOR DETERMINANT OF
SURVIVAL IN PHYCOMYCOSIS?:
A. Total dose of amphotericin B of 4000 mg
B. Early diagnosis
C. Use of potassium iodide
D. Enucleation of the eye
E. Antibiotic treatment of suppurative complications
Ref. Battock, D.J., Grausz, H., Bobrousky, M., et al: Alternate
Day Amphotericin B Therapy in the Treatment of Rhinocerebral
Phycomycosis (Mucormycosis). Ann Intern Med, 68:122, 1968.

CASE HISTORY (QUESTIONS 1088-1089)
A 22 year-old man undergoing pre-transplant hemodialysis develops
pain and tenderness at the site of his dialysis shunt   Smear of exudate
from the tubing shows only Gram positive microcci.

1088.   PRIOR TO CULTURE REPORT AND ANTIBIOTIC SENSITIVITY
TESTING, WHICH ANTIBIOTIC WOULD YOU SELECT TO INITIATE
THERAPY?:
A. Penicillin G
B. Ampicillin
C. Methicillin
D. Chloramphenicol

1089.   THE DOSE OF WHICH OF THE ABOVE ANTIBIOTICS WOULD BE
SIGNIFICANTLY AFFECTED BY HEMODIALYSIS?:
A. Penicillin G
B. Ampicillin
C. Methicillin
D. Chloramphenicol
Ref. Bulger, R.J., Petersdorf, R.G.: Antimicrobial Therapy in
Patients with Renal Insufficiency. Postgrad Med J, 47:160, 1970.

CASE HISTORY (QUESTIONS 1090-1093)
A premature infant developed a fever of 40°C, leukocytosis, and meningismus. The cerebrospinal fluid contained 4,600 cells, 85% of which were polymorphonuclear leukocytes. The cerebrospinal fluid glucose concentration was 25 mg% (Blood 96 mg%). The protein concentration was 340 mg%.

1090. AFTER OBTAINING CULTURES OF BLOOD AND CEREBROSPINAL FLUID, WHICH OF THE FOLLOWING ANTIBIOTIC REGIMENS WOULD BE APPROPRIATE?:
A. Penicillin 175,000 units/kg/day by intravenous route
B. Ampicillin 250 mg/kg/day by intravenous route plus Kanamycin 10 mg/kg/day by intramuscular route plus chloramphenicol 50 mg/kg/day by IV route
C. Penicillin 175,000 units/kg/day by intramuscular route
D. Ampicillin 250 mg/kg/day by intravenous route

1091. THE INITIAL CULTURE OF CEREBROSPINAL FLUID WAS EXAMINED 18 HOURS LATER AND FOUND TO CONTAIN A DIPHTHEROID-LIKE AEROBIC ORGANISM PRODUCING BETA HEMOLYSIS. THIS ORGANISM IS MOST LIKELY:
A. Corynebacterium acne
B. Corynebacterium diphtheriae
C. Listeria monocytogenes
D. Atypical pneumococcus
E. Corynebacterium equii

1092. ALL OF THE FOLLOWING ARE CAUSED BY THIS ORGANISM, EXCEPT:
A. Miliary granulomatosis
B. Typhoidal illness
C. Endocarditis
D. Perihepatitis
E. Oculoglandular inflammation

1093. ALL OF THE FOLLOWING STATEMENTS CONCERNING INFECTION BY THIS ORGANISM ARE CORRECT, EXCEPT:
A. Females are more commonly affected than males
B. The organism is commonly susceptible to ampicillin
C. Gram's stain of infected cerebrospinal fluid is usually negative
D. The meningitis caused by the organism is not distinctive clinically
Ref. Lavetter, A., Leedom, J.N., Mathies, A.W., et al: Meningitis due to Listeria Monocytogenes. New Eng J Med, 285:598, 1971.

CASE HISTORY (QUESTIONS 1094-1096)
A 66 year-old housewife developed fever, nausea, vomiting and
diarrhea, and was hospitalized with a fever of 40°C. Several blood
cultures contained Salmonella san diego. After 10 days of therapy
with oral and parenteral chloramphenicol succinate she was afebrile
and was discharged. Two weeks later she developed lower lumbar
pain. Spinal X-rays showed minimal vertebral osteoarthritis. The
pain became more intense and nocturnal fever appeared. Two months
after the initial hospitalization she was readmitted for investigation of
the pain.

1094. WHICH OF THE FOLLOWING WOULD BE MOST LIKELY TO IDENTIFY
       THE SOURCE OF THE PAIN?:
       A. Hemoglobin electrophoresis
       B. Cholecystogram
       C. Barium enema
       D. Lumbar spinal X-ray laminography
       E. IVP

1095. PARTIAL DESTRUCTION OF L-5 WITH COLLAPSE OF THE DISC
       SPACE IS IDENTIFIED. WHICH OF THE FOLLOWING PROCEDURES
       WOULD BE INDICATED NEXT IN IDENTIFYING THE ETIOLOGY?:
       A. Gastric cytology
       B. Blood culture
       C. Urine culture
       D. Cerebrospinal fluid culture
       E. Hemoglobin electrophoresis

1096. WHICH OF THE FOLLOWING TREATMENT PROGRAMS RESULT IN
       ARTHRODESIS WITH THE LEAST COMPLICATIONS?:
       A. 30-60 days of antibiotic therapy plus 2-3 weeks of bed rest
       B. 30-60 days of antibiotic therapy plus breast to knee cast for
           2-4 months
       C. Breast to knee cast for 4-6 months
       D. Operative verebral fusion
       E. Operative vertebral fusion plus 4-6 months of antibiotic therapy
       Ref. Jordan, M.C., Kirby, W.M.M.: Pyogenic Vertebral Osteomyelitis.
       Arch Intern Med, 128:405, 1971.

CASE HISTORY (QUESTIONS 1097-1099)
A 32 year-old woman (gravida 4, para 1, abortions 3) was admitted with
chills, fever, and prostration. One day previously she had passed a
catheter into the uterus to induce abortion. The uterus was tender.
Bacteroides sp. were cultured from the blood.

1097. WHICH OF THE FOLLOWING IS THE MOST APPROPRIATE THERAPY?:
       A. Steroid administation   D. Culdoscopy
       B. Hypothermia   E. Abdominal paracentesis
       C. Uterine curettage

1098. THE MOST COMMON ASSOCIATED OBJECTIVE PHYSICAL FINDING
       WOULD BE:
       A. Shock
       B. Tender adnexae
       C. Lower abdominal tenderness
       D. Massive uterine bleeding
       E. Foul cervical discharge

1099. BACTEROIDES BACTEREMIA IS MOST OFTEN ACCOMPANIED BY
       BACTEREMIA INVOLVING:
       A. S. albus
       B. Non-hemolytic aerobic streptococci
       C. Clsotridium species
       D. Group A beta hemolytic streptococci
       E. Microaerophilic-anaerobic streptococci
       Ref. Pearson, H. E. , Anderson, G. V. : Bacteroides Infections and
       Pregnancy. Obs Gyn, 35:31, 1970.

       CASE HISTORY (QUESTIONS 1100-1103)
       A 26 year-old man developed sneezing, headache and malaise
       followed in 18 hours by sore throat, rhinorrhea, and nasal congestion.

1100. THE MOST COMMON ASSOCIATED OBJECTIVE FINDING WOULD BE:
       A. Cough   D. Serous otitis media
       B. Fever   E. Nasal discharge
       C. Erythematous eruption

1101. THIS SYNDROME MAY BE CAUSED BY:
       A. Rhinovirus   D. Coronavirus
       B. Influenza virus, Type A   E. All of the above
       C. Echovirus

1102. BACTERIOLOGIC CULTURE OF THE THROAT WOULD BE EXPECTED
       TO SHOW:
       A. Corynebacterium diphtheriae
       B. No change from normal
       C. Candida albicans
       D. Hemophilus influenzae
       E. None of the above

1103. OF MANY SUGGESTED DRUGS, THE FOLLOWING IS USUALLY
       EFFECTIVE:
       A. Large doses of vitamin C   D. Tranquilizers
       B. Antihistaminics   E. None of the above
       C. Bioflavonoids
       Ref. Jackson, G. G. : The Common Cold in Textbook of Medicine,
       Ed, Beeson, P. B. , McDermott, W. , W. B. Saunders Co. , Philadelphia,
       1971, p. 361.

       CASE HISTORY (QUESTIONS 1104-1106)
       A 57 year-old turkey farmer presented complaining of a slowly
       progressive febrile illness of 14 days duration. The illness began with
       malaise, anorexia, severe myalgia and unremitting fever, initially
       $38^{o}C$ but rising to $40^{o}C$ during the week. Cough productive of small
       amounts of blood-streaked mucus began on the 5th day of the illness.
       A macular rash was noted on the chest the day of examiniation.
       Epistaxis appeared on the second day of the illness. He had been
       nauseated and vomited frequently throughout the 10 day period. On
       exam: T-$40.5^{o}C$; P-48/min; R-36/min; BP 150/80

1104. WHICH OF THE FOLLOWING PHYSICAL FINDINGS IS MOST LIKELY?:
       A. Auscultatory findings of pneumonic consolidation
       B. Arthritis
       C. Jaundice
       D. Splenomegaly
       E. Pleural friction rub

1105.   WHICH OF THE FOLLOWING PROCEDURES WOULD MOST LIKELY
         BE DIAGNOSTIC AT THE TIME OF EXAMINATION?:
         A. Chest X-ray
         B. Determination of complement fixing antibody titer to appropriate
             antigens
         C. Determination of antibody to Salmonella "O" antigens
         D. Frei test
         E. Bone marrow biopsy

1106.   THERAPY SHOULD BE INSTITUTED USING:
         A. Chloramphenicol 500 mgm p. o. q. 6h
         B. Penicillin 600, 000 units I. M. q 12 h
         C. Tetracycline 250 mgm po q6h
         D. Penicillin 600, 000 units I. M. q 12 h plus tetracycline 250 mgm po q6h
         E. None of the above
         Ref. Rogers, D. E.: Psittacosis in Textbook of Medicine, Ed, Beeson,
         P. B., McDermott, W., W. B. Saunders Co., Philadelphia, 1971, p. 374.

CASE HISTORY (QUESTIONS 1107-1109)
A 12 year-old boy developed pain in the right lumbar region at the site
of trauma sustained 24 hours previously. Over the next 7 days he
developed malaise, increasing pain in the right lumbar area, and
chills. On examination: T-40.3°C; P-118/min; R26/min; BP110/70.
A warm tender mass which was red but not fluctuant extended
from the midscapular paravertebrally over the iliac crest. The
remainder of the physical examination was negative. WBC 22, 300/cu mm.

1107.   NEEDLE ASPIRATION OF THE MASS WOULD BE EXPECTED TO
         YIELD:
         A. Bacteroides species
         B. Clostridium perfringens
         C. Arizona species
         D. Staphylococcus aureus
         E. Negative bacteriologic culture

1108.   AN ELECTROMYOGRAM OF MUSCLES IN THIS AREA WOULD SHOW:
         A. Myopathic features   D. Recruitment
         B. Defibrillation   E. Normal pattern
         C. Myasthenic features

1109.   WHICH OF THE FOLLOWING ARE ALSO FEATURES OF THIS
         DISEASE?:
         A. Single abscesses are more common than multiple abscesses
         B. Blood cultures are usually positive
         C. The commonest sites of abscess formation are distal leg muscles
         D. Healing usually produces extensive residua
         E. Local lymph nodes are almost always enlarged
         Ref. Altrocchi, P. H.: Spontaneous Bacterial Myositis. JAMA,
         217:819, 1971.

CASE HISTORY (QUESTIONS 1110-1113)
A 45 year-old spinster sustained deep bite wounds of the right finger
incident to separating two fighting cats. Within 24 hours there was
cellulitis of the finger, severe throbbing pain, erythema of the forearm,
and epitrochlear lymphadenitis. T 39.2°C; R-12/min; P-110/min;
BP 120/78. Smear of pus from the lesion demonstrated small
gram-negative coccobacillary bacteria.

1110. WHICH OF THE FOLLOWING MEDIA WOULD <u>NOT</u> SUPPORT THE
       GROWTH OF THIS ORGANISM?:
       A. Trypticase soy agar
       B. 5% human blood agar
       C. MacConkey agar
       D. 5% sheep blood agar
       E. Brain heart infusion broth

1111. WHICH OF THE FOLLOWING INFECTIONS HAS ALSO BEEN
       ASSOCIATED WITH THIS ORGANISM?:
       A. Bronchiectasis   D. Septic arthritis
       B. Chorioamnionitis   E. All of the above
       C. Meningitis

1112. CULTURAL CHARACTERISTICS OF THIS ORGANISM INCLUDE:
       A. Alpha hemolysis
       B. Optimum growth at 37°C
       C. No growth on salmonella-shigella agar
       D. Oxidase positive
       E. All of the above

1113. MOST STRAINS OF THIS ORGANISM ARE RESISTANT TO:
       A. Tetracycline   D. Erythromycin
       B. Penicillin   E. None of the above
       C. Bacitracin
       Ref. DeBoer, R.G. , Dumler, M. : Pasturella Multocida Infections.
       Amer J Clin Path, 40:339, 1963. Strand, C.L. , Helfman, L. :
       Pasturella Multocida Chorioamnionitis Associated with Premature
       Delivery and Neonatal Sepsis and Death. Amer J Clin Path, 55:713,
       1971.

CASE HISTORY (QUESTIONS 1114-1117)
A 24 year-old merchant seaman was admitted to an East Coast Hospital.
His ship had made calls in Nicaragua and several other Central
American ports the week before he experienced the abrupt onset of
diarrhea and abdominal pain. He had eaten food at several of the ports
of call. On admission he was acutely ill, dehydrated, and febrile
(40.2°C). The abdomen was soft and tender in both lower quadrants.
Profuse watery diarrhea containing mucus and blood was noted. The
rectal mucosa was hyperemic and friable, but no ulcers were seen.
WBC 18,000/cu mm.

1114. STOOL CULTURES YIELDED AN INTESTINAL PATHOGEN. WHICH
       OF THE FOLLOWING IS MOST LIKELY?:
       A. Salmonella typhimurium
       B. Shigella dysenteriae
       C. Providence sp.
       D. Enteropathic E. coli
       E. Giardia lamblia

1115.   THE RESPONSIBLE ORGANISM WOULD GROW BEST ON WHICH OF
        THE FOLLOWING DURING PRIMARY ISOLATION?:
        A. Chocolate agar
        B. 5% sheep's blood agar
        C. Salmonella-Shigella agar
        D. Tergitol 7 agar (T7T)
        E. Thioglycollate broth

1116.   THE ORGANISM COULD BE EXPECTED TO BE RESISTANT TO
        WHICH OF THE FOLLOWING ANTIBIOTICS?:
        A. Tetracycline   D. Nalidixic acid
        B. Kanamycin   E. Ampicillin
        C. Cephalothin

1117.   ALL OF THE FOLLOWING STATEMENTS CONCERNING THIS INFECTIO
        ARE TRUE, EXCEPT:
        A. Antibiotic sensitivity testing of the organism is necessary
        B. The presentation may be indistinguishable from ulcerative colitis
        C. Antibiotic therapy is not mandatory
        D. Most strains of this organism are resistant to chloramphenicol
        E. Blood cultures may contain the organism
        Ref. Counts, G.W., Nitzkin, J.L., Hennekens, C.H., Ehrenkranz,
        N.J.: Shiga Bacillus Dysentery Acquired in Nicaragua. Arch Intern Med,
        128:582, 1971.

        CASE HISTORY (QUESTIONS 1118-1121)
        An 18 year-old man was admitted to a hospital in New Mexico
        because of severe malaise, shaking chills, dizziness, headache, and
        extremely painful swelling in the right groin. He was employed by
        the Parks Department in clearing brush from new campsites and had
        noted numerous bites over the lower extremities. On examination he was
        oriented but acutely ill; T-104° orally; BP 120/70; P-122; R-20.
        The only positive physical findings were conjunctivitis and a 3 cm
        erythematous mass in the right groin below the inguinal ligament.
        The chest X-ray was normal.

1118.   WHICH OF THE FOLLOWING WOULD MOST QUICKLY IDENTIFY AN
        ORGANISM RESPONSIBLE FOR THIS DISEASE?:
        A. Blood culture
        B. Buffy coat smear Gram's stain
        C. Gram's stain of aspirate from the mass
        D. Giemsa stain of aspirate from the mass
        E. Culture of aspirate from the mass

1119.   IF A STAIN OF THE ASPIRATE FROM THE MASS WAS PERFORMED
        AND SHOWED BIPOLAR STAINING RODS, WHICH OF THE FOLLOWING
        ANTIBIOTICS WOULD YOU ADMINISTER?:
        A. Streptomycin
        B. Penicillin and chloramphenicol
        C. Kanamycin
        D. Streptomycin and tetracycline
        E. Tetracycline

1120.   THERAPY SHOULD BE CONTINUED FOR WHAT LENGTH OF TIME?:
        A. 10-14 days
        B. 3 weeks after defervesence
        C. 7 days
        D. 6 weeks
        E. None of the above

1121.   WHICH OF THE FOLLOWING ANIMALS ARE INVOLVED IN THE
        TRANSMISSION OF THIS DISEASE?:
        A. Squirrels   D. Dogs
        B. Rats   E. All of the above
        C. Cats
        Ref. Palmer, D. L. , Kisch, A. L. , Williams, R. C. , Jr. , et al:
        Clinical Features of Plague in the United States: The 1969-1970
        Epidemic. J Inf Dis, 124:367, 1971.

        CASE HISTORY (QUESTIONS 1122-1124)
        A 53 year-old man with chronic bronchitis and emphysema developed
        a sore throat, sniffles, and exacerbation of his cough, usually
        productive of 30-40 cc of white viscid sputum. Because of increasing
        shortness of breath he was hospitalized in the respiratory care unit.
        On admission: T-100.5°F; R-28/min; P-108   regular; BP 150/90.
        The sputum contained many leukocytes plus both gram-positive and
        negative cocci. Ampicillin, 500 mgm orally, was administered every
        6 hours in addition to an intensive bronchial toilet. On the 3rd
        hospital day his temperature was normal but he remainded dyspneic.
        On the fourth hospital day the sputum culture showed a few alpha
        hemolytic streptococci but contained a heavy growth of Enterobacter
        hafniae.

1122.   TO WHICH OF THE FOLLOWING ANTIBIOTICS WOULD YOU
        EXPECT E. HAFNIAE TO BE SENSITIVE?: (AGAR DILUTION
        TECHNIQUE)?:
        A. Ampicillin   D. Cephalothin
        B. Penicillin   E. Cephalexin
        C. Gentamicin

1123.   WHICH OF THE FOLLOWING IS NOT A CULTURAL CHARACTERISTIC
        OF MOST STRAINS OF ENTEROBACTER HAFNIAE?:
        A. Glucose fermentation
        B. Hydrogen sulfide production
        C. Nitrate reduction
        D. Motility at 35°C
        E. Resistance to ampicillin

1124.   WHICH THERAPEUTIC APPROACH WOULD YOU RECOMMEND IN
        VIEW OF THE PRESENCE OF E. HAFNIAE IN THE SPUTUM OF
        THIS PATIENT?:
        A. Continue ampicillin, add gentamicin 5 mg/kg/day 1M in 3 doses
        B. Stop ampicillin, begin cephalothin 2 gm IV every 6 hours
        C. Stop ampicillin
        D. Stop ampicillin, begin carbenicillin 500 mgm/kg/day IV in 4 doses
            plus gentamicin as in A (above)
        E. None of the above
        Ref. Washington, J. A. , Birk, R. J. , Ritts, R. E. , Jr.: Bacteriologic
        and Epidemiologic Characteristics of Enterobacter Hafniae and
        Enterobacter Liquefaciens. J Inf Dis, 124:379, 1971.

CASE HISTORY (QUESTIONS 1125-1127)

A 25 year-old woman was hospitalized for migratory polyarthritis of
3 days duration. She noted the abrupt onset of swelling and erythema
of the right elbow, left shoulder and both knees. Three days prior
to the arthritis she had noted a profuse whitish vaginal discharge.
On the day of admission, pustules surrounded by erythema had
appeared on both hands and forearms. She had been treated twice for
gonorrhea in the 7 weeks prior to admission. On examination:
BP 110/80; P-108/min; R19/min; T-38.2°C orally. There was a
maculopapular eruption over both knees and tender pustules over
both forearms. All the joints noted above were tender, hot, and
swollen. Aside from the purulent endocervical discharge, the
examination of the genitalia and pelvis were normal. Laboratory data:
WBC 10, 200 (65% PMN 5% bands); ESR 90 mm/hr; cultures of endo-
cervix, rectum, and blood all contained Neisseria gonorrhoeae;
VDRL negative. The patient is not allergic to penicillin.

1125.   IN ADDITION TO ARTHRITIS, OTHER COMPLICATIONS OF
        GONORRHEA ARE:
        A. Meningitis   D. Endocarditis
        B. Ophthalmitis   E. All of the above
        C. Perihepatis

1126.   WHICH OF THE FOLLOWING IS APPROPRIATE THERAPY FOR
        THIS WOMAN?:
        A. Aqueous penicillin G procaine 4.8 million units IM
        B. Benzathine penicillin 4.8 million units IM
        C. Aqueous penicillin G procaine 600, 000 units IM q 12 h for 5 days
        D. Aqueous penicillin G 8-10 million units per day for 8-10 days
        E. Tetracycline 1.5 gm per day orally for 30 days

1127.   HOST IMMUNITY TO REINFECTION GONORRHEA LASTS FOR WHAT
        PERIOD OF TIME AFTER A PREVIOUS ATTACK OF GONORRHEA?:
        A. Days
        B. Weeks
        C. Months
        D. Years
        Ref. Caldwell, J. G. , Wessler, S. , Avroli, L. V.: Current Therapy
        of Gonorrhea. JAMA, 218:714, 1971.

CASE HISTORY (QUESTIONS 1128-1129)

A 26 year-old man is referred to you by the local health authorities
because a woman with whom he had intercourse 3 times in the past
12 days has been found to have infectious syphilis. In the past 24
hours, he has developed severe dysuria and a purulent urethral
discharge. Gram's stain of the discharge shows gram-negative
intracellular diplococci. Otherwise, close inspection of the genitalia
reveals no abnormalities. There have been no other infectious
contacts. He is not allergic to penicillin and the VDRL is negative.

1128.   WHICH TREATMENT REGIMEN WOULD YOU SELECT?:
        A. Aqueous procaine penicillin G, 2.4 million units IM
        B. Aqueous procaine penicillin G, 2.4 million units IM plus 2.4
            million units of benzathine penicillin IM
        C. Aqueous procaine penicillin G, 4.8 million units IM plus
            benzathine penicillin 4.8 million units IM
        D. Tetracycline phosphate, 3.0 gms orally
        E. Tetracycline phosphate. 1.5 gms orally

1129. THE OBSERVED EFFICACY OF THE PREFERRED REGIMEN (IN THE QUESTION ABOVE) FOR THE TREATMENT OF GONORRHEA WHILE ABORTING INCUBATING SYPHILIS IS:

A. 10%   D. 27%
B. 50%   E. 0%
C. 100%

Ref. Schroeter, A. L. , Turner, R. H. , Lucas, J. B. , Brown, W. J. : Therapy for Incubating Syphilis; Effectiveness of Gonorrhea Treatment. JAMA, 218:711, 1971.

CASE HISTORY (QUESTION 1130)
A 64 year-old diabetic and hypertensive man is admitted with signs of occlusion of the right middle cerebral artery. A lumbar puncture is performed. Although the last tube obtained is clear, there are 30 erythrocytes/cu mm in this tube. The VDRL performed using fluid from this tube is 1:4. The peripheral blood VDRL titer is 1:8.

1130. WHAT IS YOUR INTERPRETATION OF THESE FINDINGS?:

A. The VDRL in the spinal fluid is caused by contamination by VDRL positive blood
B. The spinal fluid VDRL probably represents a truly reactive CSF serology
C. The spinal fluid FTA-ABS test would be expected to be negative
D. The spinal fluid reactions are of no value and cannot be interpreted

Ref. Izzat, N. N. , Bartruff, J. K. , Glicksman, J. M. , et al: Validity of the VDRL test on Cerebrospinal Fluid Contaminated by Blood. Brit J Ven Dis, 47:162, 1971.

CASE HISTORY (QUESTIONS 1131-1133)
A 65 year-old woman was hospitalized with a 5-day history of intermittent chills with fever. Previously, she had received transfusion therapy and azothioprine for red cell aplasia. On the day of admission she complained of malaise, frontal headache, and arthralgia. There was no skin rash, diarrhea, cough, or recent dental or surgical procedures. She lived on a cattle-raising farm in Mississippi but denied close contact with animals and had seen no abortions. For 3 weeks she had been eating blended raw beef liver which she thought might improve her anemia. On examination: BP 140/90; P-112/min; R-18/min; T-39ºC orally. On physical examination the head, neck, heart, and chest were normal. The liver was palpable 3 cm below the costal margin and was firm and tender. The neurologic examination was normal. No arthritis was noted. Three blood cultures obtained on admission yielded Vibrio fetus.

1131. THE EPIDEMIOLOGY OF THIS INFECTION INCLUDES:

A. Direct contact with infected animals
B. Venereal transmission among humans
C. Contamination of food and water
D. Placental transfer or exposure at delivery
E. All of the above

1132. WHICH OF THE FOLLOWING UNDERLYING CONDITIONS IS MOST FREQUENTLY ASSOCIATED WITH VIBRIO sp. INFECTIONS OF MAN?:

A. Sarcoma   D. Sarcoid
B. Leukemia   E. Induced abortion
C. Alcoholism

1133.   THE ORGANISM IS USUALLY RESISTANT TO:
        A. Tetracycline   D. Kanamycin
        B. Penicillin   E. Ampicillin
        C. Chloramphenicol
        Ref. Soonattrakul, W., Andersen, B., Bryner, J.H.: Raw Liver as a
        Possible source of Vibrio Fetus Septicemia in Man. Amer J Med Sci,
        261:245, 1971.

        CASE HISTORY (QUESTIONS 1134-1137)
        A 42 year-old woman was hospitalized because of low grade fever,
        cough productive of yellow sputum, right-sided pleuritic pain, and
        dyspnea of 3 days duration. There was no history of alcoholism,
        smoking, or chronic lung disease. She had adult onset diabetes
        mellitus, well controlled with 500 mgm tolbutamide t.i.d. On
        examination: R-56/min; P-140/min; T-40.5°C; BP 120/70 mmHg.
        Bilateral coarse rales were heard at the right base. There was a
        friction rub heard in the right base. WBC 14,800 (82% PMN 18% lymph);
        BUN 12; Blood glucose 184. Chest X-ray showed a right lower lobe
        segmental pneumonia and a moderate pleural effusion on the right.
        Sputum cultures contained H. influenzae in addition to normal flora.

1134.   TO ESTABLISH THE ETIOLOGY OF THE PNEUMONIA, THE MOST
        APPROPRIATE PROCEDURE IS:
        A. Repeat sputum culture
        B. Acid fast stain of the sputum
        C. Blood culture
        D. Cold agglutinin titer
        E. KOH examination of sputum

1135.   ASSUMING THAT THE NEXT DAY 3 BLOOD CULTURES CONTAIN
        H. INFLUENZAE TYPE B, ONE COUD ASSUME:
        A. H. influenzae is rarely pathogenic for adults, so another organism
            must also be present
        B. The strain of H. influenzae isolated is probably non-encapsulated,
            since these are the invasive strains
        C. The organism in the blood and sputum are different strains of
            H. influenzae
        D. The patient probably has a low or non-existent titer of anticapsular
            antibody
        E. None of the above

1136.   WHICH OF THE FOLLOWING IS CHARACTERISTIC OF PNEUMONIA
        CAUSED BY BOTH D. PNEUMONIAE AND H. INFLUENZA?:
        A. Capacity to cause segmental pneumonia
        B. Capacity to cause lobar pneumonia
        C. Production of a pleural effusion
        D. Bacteremia
        E. All of the above

1137.   WHICH OF THE FOLLOWING LABORATORY PROCEDURES WOULD
        HELP TO IDENTIFY THIS STRAIN OF H. INFLUENZAE AS
        PATHOGENIC?:
        A. Satellite growth around S. aureus
        B. Capsular typing
        C. Colonial appearance
        D. Hemolysis
        E. Ability to grow on chocolate agar
        Ref. Quintiliani, R., Hymans, P.J.: The Association of Bacteremic
        Haemophilus Influenzae Pneumonia in Adults with Typable Strains.
        Amer J Med, 50:781, 1971.

CASE HISTORY (QUESTIONS 1138-1139)
A 23 year-old patient consults a physician at a student health center
because of fever and arthritis. Gram-negative diplococci
are seen in joint fluid, and N. gonorrhoeae is obtained from several
blood cultures.

1138.   WHICH OF THE FOLLOWING CLINICAL CHARACTERISTICS WOULD
         BE MOST NEARLY CORRECT?:
         A.   Patient is more likely to be a woman than a man
         B.   The joint most likely to be involved is the hip joint
         C.   The white count (in the absence of prior antibiotic therapy) is most
              likely to be below 5000/cu mm.
         D.   Almost all patients are febrile
         E.   History of sexual contact is nearly universal

1139.   WHICH OF THE SYNOVIALYSES BELOW WOULD FIT THE EXPECTED
         FINDINGS?:

	Leukocyte count	Protein gm/100 ml	Mucin clot
A.	50,000	5.8	good
B.	50,000	5.8	poor
C.	50,000	1.0	good
D.	100	1.0	good
E.	100	1.2	poor

Ref. Cooke, C. L., Owen, D. S., Jr., Irby, R., et al: Gonococcal
Arthritis. JAMA, 217:204, 1971.

CASE HISTORY (QUESTION 1140)
A 21 year-old medical student is referred to the health service because
a routine chest X-ray revealed an infiltrate in the posterior aspect of
the left upper lobe. One year ago the chest X-ray was normal. There
are no symptoms and physical examination is normal. Six months
ago the reaction to 5 TU of PPD-S injected intradermally was negative.
Four intradermal skin tests give the following results at 48 hours:

	Antigen	Mm induration
1.	PPD-S	5 x 6
2.	PPD-B (Battey)	18 x 16
3.	PPD-G (Scotochromogen)	15 x 12
4.	PPD-Y (Kansasii)	20 x 21

1140.   WHAT CAN YOU CONCLUDE FROM THESE DATA?:
         A.   The antigen homologous to the infecting organism is PPD-Y
         B.   The disease is probably not due to M. tuberculosis hominis
         C.   The disease is likely to be caused by M. tuberculosis hominis
         D.   These tests identify the Battery bacillus as the responsible organism
         Ref. Edwards, P. Q.: Significance of the Tuberculin Test Today.
         Clin Notes Resp Dis, 8:1, 1969.

CASE HISTORY (QUESTION 1141)

A 28 year-old black woman with documented pulmonary sarcoidosis of
6 years duration presents because of cough not productive of sputum.
The reaction to intradermal PPD-S (5TU) was known to be negative
on a number of occasions. The chest X-ray is stable as is the physical
examination. A repeat intradermal test using 5 TU of PPD-S yields
an area of induration 12 x 14 mm at 48 hours.

1141.   YOUR INTERPRETATION IS:
        A. The positive PPD represents recovery from sarcoid
        B. Patient should be retested using 1 TU
        C. Patient probably does not have active tuberculosis
        D. Patient probably has tuberculosis superimposed on sarcoid
        E. None of the above
        Ref. Chusid, E. L., Shah, R., Siltzbach, L. E.: Tuberculin
        Testing During the Course of Sarcoidosis in 350 Patients. Amer Rev
        Resp Dis, 104:13, 1971.

CASE HISTORY (QUESTIONS 1142-1145)

A 42 year-old woman had been under treatment for culturally
confirmed cavitary pulmonary tuberculosis for 7 months when she
developed anorexia, cough, and weight loss. Repeat X-rays revealed
a mass within a persistent cavity in the right upper lobe. The mass
had not been seen 4 months earlier.

1142.   WHICH OF THE FOLLOWING ORGANISMS WOULD BE EXPECTED
        TO BE PRESENT IN HER SPUTUM?:
        A. M. tuberculosis   D. Candida sp.
        B. H. capsulatum   E. None of the above
        C. Aspergillus sp.

1143.   EXAMINATION OF HER SERUM WOULD MOST PROBABLY SHOW:
        A. Positive precipitating antibodies to aspergillus
        B. Negative precipitating antibodies to aspergillus
        C. Diagnostic titers of complement fixing antibodies to H. capsulatum
        D. None of the above

1144.   OF THE FOLLOWING, THE MOST IMPORTANT DIAGNOSTIC STUDY IS:
        A. Pleural biopsy   D. Tomography of the chest
        B. Lung biopsy   E. Tuberculin skin test
        C. Lung scan

1145.   THE MOST DANGEROUS COMPLICATION IN THIS PATIENT IS:
        A. Brain abscess   D. Pneumonia
        B. Empyema   E. Meningitis
        C. Hemoptysis
        Ref. Solit, R. W., McKeown, J. J., Smullens, S., et al: The
        Surgical Implications of Intracavitary Mycetomas (Fungus Balls).
        J Thor Cardiovasc Surg, 62:411, 1971.

CASE HISTORY (QUESTION 1146)

A 29 year-old man developed acute myeloblastic leukemia and was treated with prednisone, vincristine, methotrexate, and 6-mercapatopurine. A short remission occurred, but 2 months later the patient was hospitalized because of oral ulcerations and fever. On examination: BP 110/70; P-110; R-18; T-40°C (orally). The mouth was beefy red and a white exudate covered the palate. The remainder of the physical examination was unremarkable. Laboratory data: WBC 1400 (20% neutrophils); the bone marrow was hypoplastic; CSF-normal; smear of the oral exudate revealed budding yeasts. Candida sp were obtained from the blood.

1146.   WITH SYSTEMIC CANDIDIASIS YOU WOULD ALSO ANTICIPATE:
A. Negative tests for serum anti-candida precipitating or agglutinating antibodies
B. Positive tests for serum anti-candida precipitating or agglutinating antibodies in all cases
C. Positive tests for serum anti-candida precipitating or agglutinating antibodies in the majority of cases
D. No relation to response to treatment and titer of serum anti-candida precipitating or agglutinating antibodies
E. None of the above

Ref. Rosner, F., Gabriel, F.D., Taschdjian, C.L., et al: Serologic Diagnosis of Candidiasis in Patients with Acute Leukemia. Amer J Med, 51:54, 1971.

CASE HISTORY (QUESTIONS 1147-1149)

A 19 year-old heroin addict was admitted to a hospital because of right-sided low back pain. Physical examination: T(oral) 99.2°F; BP 130/65; R-12/min; Pulse 80/min. The heart and lungs were normal. The liver and spleen were not enlarged. There were no petachiae or splinter hemorrhages. The right sacroiliac joint area was exquisitely tender. The following X-rays were normal - chest, abdomen, barium enema, IVP, upper GI series, l-s spine. An intermediate PPD showed 3 mm induration at 48 hours. ESR = 39 mm/hr; WBC = 18,000 cu mm (90% neutrophils). During an 8-day course, fever to 101° and persistent back pain were noted. Repeat X-rays showed periosteal elevation at the L 3-4 interspace.

1147.   WHICH OF THE FOLLOWING DIAGNOSTIC PROCEDURES SHOULD BE PERFORMED NEXT?:
A. Tomograms of L3-4 area
B. Additional blood cultures
C. Second strength PPD
D. Surgical exploration of L3-4

1148.   WHICH OF THE FOLLOWING ORGANISMS WOULD NOT BE EXPECTED TO PRODUCE THIS LESION?:
A. Pseudomonas aeruginosa
B. Candida stellatoidea
C. Gr A beta hemolytic streptococci
D. Staphylococcus aureus

1149.   WHICH OF THE FOLLOWING CLINICAL CONDITIONS IS MOST
        LIKELY TO BE ASSOCIATED?:
        A. Tuberculosis
        B. Hepatitis
        C. Endocarditis
        D. Brain abscess
        Ref. Holzman, R. S. , Bishko, F. : Osteomyelitis in Heroin Addicts.
        Ann Intern Med, 75:693, 1971.

        CASE HISTORY (QUESTIONS 1150-1152)
        A 24 year-old laborer sustained multiple bullet wounds to the abdomen
        during a tavern brawl. Devitalized bowel was removed at surgery and
        a colostomy performed. On the fourth postoperative day fecal
        material began to drain from the wound. An entero-cutaneous fistula
        and a fistula between the small bowel and descending colon were
        demonstrated by X-ray. In order to maintain fluid balance, 5%
        amino-acid solution in combination with fructose and alcohol were
        infused for 14 days through a right subclavian catheter which was
        inspected daily. The catheter wound was dressed with neomycin-
        polymyxin-bacitracin ointment daily. On the 14th day of hyper-
        alimentation, he developed fever of 40.6°C accompanied by shaking
        chills. Blood cultures yielded Candida albicans. A millipore
        membrane filter was in place in the infusion line during therapy.

1150.   WHICH OF THE FOLLOWING WOULD BE MOST LIKELY TO ALSO
        YIELD C. ALBICANS ON CULTURES?:
        A. The hyperalimentation fluid
        B. Tip of intravenous catheter
        C. The neomycin-polymyxin-bacitracin ointment
        D. The millipore filter

1151.   NEXT TO C. ALBICANS, WHICH OF THE FOLLOWING IS MOST
        LIKELY TO CAUSE SEPSIS UNDER THESE CIRCUMSTANCES?:
        A. T. glabrata
        B. C. neoformans
        C. Mucor species
        D. N. asteroides

1152.   WHICH OF THE FOLLOWING UNDERLYING DISEASES WOULD YOU
        ANTICIPATE FINDING IN THIS PATIENT?:
        A. Hodgkin's disease
        B. Leukemia
        C. Polyarteritis nodosa
        D. Aplastic anemia
        E. None of the above
        Ref. Curry, C. R. , Quie, P. G. : Fungal Septicemia in Patients
        Receiving Parenteral Hyperalimentation. New Eng J Med, 285:1221,
        1971.

CASE HISTORY (QUESTIONS 1153-1155)
A 35 year-old man developed a macular papular rash 12 hours after
a beach outing during which he waded into the sea to collect clams.
He also ate several raw clams. The next day he vomited and had
5 loose stools. That day he noted the rash was becoming darker.
On examination: T-40.3°C; P-118/min; BP 130/70; R-16/min. There
was a papular hemorrhagic rash over the entire body except the face.
Several large vesicles were present on the lower extremities. Gram's
stain of the fluid showed a pleomorphic gram-negative rod.

1153. THE MOST LIKELY ETIOLOGIC AGENT IS:
A. Hepatitis virus   D. P. aeruginosa
B. R. rickettsii   E. Salmonella sp.
C. Vibrio parahemolyticus

1154. WHICH OF THE FOLLOWING IS NOT A CHARACTERISTIC OF
VIBRIO sp. PRODUCING DISEASE IN MAN?:
A. Motility   D. Hemolytic
B. Negative oxidase test   E. Halophilic
C. Single polar flagellum

1155. TO WHICH OF THE FOLLOWING ANTIBIOTICS IS V. PARAHEMO-
LYTICUS USUALLY SENSITIVE?:
A. Penicillin   D. Bacitracin
B. Polymyxin B   E. Erythromycin
C. Polymyxin E
Ref. Roland, F. P.: Vibrio Parahemolyticus. Clin Med, 78:26, 1971.

CASE HISTORY (QUESTIONS 1156-1158)
A 23 year-old man suddenly developed chilly sensations, malaise,
and felt "feverish" on the 6th day of a hiking trip through mountains in
Colorado. He had removed numerous ticks in the previous days,
although none were engorged. After 2 days of headache and backache,
he felt much better for 2 days, but consulted a physician when all his
previous symptoms recurred. Examination: BP 110/82; P-100;
R-10; T-39. 3°C orally. The physical exam was within the normal
range. No rash or splenomegaly was noted.

1156. THE MOST PROBABLE ETIOLOGY IS:
A. Plague
B. Rocky Mountain spotted fever
C. Colorado tick fever
D. Influenza
E. Relapsing fever

1157. THE MOST LIKELY LABORATORY ABNORMALITY IS:
A. Marked leukopenia   D. Hematuria
B. Leukemoid response   E. Borrelemia
C. Eosinophilia

1158. TREATMENT SHOULD CONSIST OF:
A. Penicillin and streptomycin
B. Supportive care
C. Tetracycline
D. Chloramphenicol
E. Streptomycin and tetracycline
Ref. Meiklejohn, G.: Colorado Tick Fever in Textbook of Medicine.
Beeson, P. B., McDermott, W., (Ed), W. B. Saunders Co., Philadelphia,
1971, p. 432.

CASE HISTORY (QUESTION 1159)
A 26 year-old diabetic underwent an uncomplicated appendectomy
following 3 days of right lower quadrant pain and fever. The appendix
was not ruptured. No pre- or postoperative antibiotics were used.
He was afebrile postoperatively until the third day when fever to
40°C orally was noted. An indwelling intravenous catheter was
removed because of thrombophlebitis at the site.

1159. IN A GROUP OF SUCH PATIENTS THE ORGANISM MOST FREQUENTLY
CULTURED FROM THE TIP OF THE INTRAVENOUS CATHETER IS:
A. Staphylococcus aureus   D. Bacteroides sp.
B. Providence sp.   E. M. polymorpha
C. Serratia sp.
Ref. Altemeier, W. A. , McDonough, J. J. , Fuller, W. D. : Third Day
Surgery Fever. Arch Surg, 103:158, 1971.

CASE HISTORY (QUESTION 1160)
An 11 year-old girl was immunized by the parenteral route with live
attenuated rubella vaccine (HPV-77 DK/12). In the ensuing 3 months
she developed recurrent moderately painful effusions of the right knee,
left elbow, and right wrist. Three months after immunization the
left knee was swollen, warm, and painful.

1160. SEROLOGIC AND VIROLOGIC SUTDIES WOULD MOST LIKELY REVEAL:
A. IgA antibodies only in the joint fluid
B. Large amount of IgM rubella antibody in the serum
C. Large amount of IgG rubella antibody in the nasopharynx
D. No IgG rubella antibodies in the serum
E. Rubella virus in the joint fluid
Ref. Ogra, P. L. , Herd, J. L. : Arthritis Associated with Induced
Rubella Infection. J Immunol, 107:810, 1971.

CASE HISTORY (QUESTIONS 1161-1163)
A 24 year-old Vietnam veteran sustained third degree burns over
55% of the body surface 2 months after discharge. After an initially
satisfactory response to therapy, he became febrile on the tenth
hospital day. On examination: BP 40/0; R-40; T-41°C (rectal);
P-135/min. The burn sites were not grossly infected. The chest
X-ray was unremarkable. His condition quickly deteriorated, and he
died 8 hours after the shock syndrome appeared. Four blood cultures
contained a gram-negative oxidase-positive motile rod which produced
no soluble pigment or hemolysis.

1161. CORRECT ANTIBIOTIC THERAPY FOR THIS INFECTION INCLUDES:
A. Kanamycin and chloramphenicol
B. Tetracycline and Kanamycin
C. Tetracycline and chloramphenicol
D. Sulfadiazine and chloramphenicol
E. Novobiocin

1162. AT AUTOPSY, WHICH OF THE FOLLOWING SYSTEMS IS LEAST
LIKELY TO BE INVOLVED BY THIS INFECTION?:
A. Lungs
B. Gastrointestinal system
C. Liver
D. Spleen
E. Kidneys

163.   CHRONIC INFECTION WITH THIS ORGANISM IS OFTEN CONFUSED WITH:

A. Pulmonary tuberculosis   D. Syphilis
B. Shigellosis   E. Schistosomiasis
C. Malaria

Ref. Howe, C., Sampath, A., Spotnitz, M.: The Pseudomallei Group:
A Review. J Inf Dis, 124:598, 1972.

CASE HISTORY (QUESTIONS 1164-1168)

A 49 year-old man with a strong history of alcoholism and biopsy-
proven cirrhosis presented to hospital complaining of diffuse abdominal
pain of three days duration. In previous outpatient visits he had been
observed to have ascites, but liver function tests (bilirubin, SGOT,
SGPT, alkaline phosphatase) 1 month earlier had been normal.
On examination: BP 132/86; R-12; T-39°C (oral); P-116/min. The
examination showed stigmata of cirrhosis which were unchanged from the
previous admission. Intellectual function had clearly deteriorated.
Laboratory findings: WBC 20,000/cu. mm (92% polymorphonuclear
leukocytes), Hgb 11.1; Urine analysis - normal; X-rays of chest -
no pneumonia or effusion; Abdominal X-rays - Normal gas pattern with
findings of ascites. Ascitic fluid was obtained with following findings:
WBC 13,000/cu. mm., sp. gr. 1.019.

1164.   CULTURES OF THE ASCITIC FLUID WOULD MOST LIKELY YIELD:

A. Klebsiella sp.   D. Citrobacter sp.
B. E. coli   E. Salmonella sp.
C. Bacteroides sp.

1165.   THE LIVER FUNCTION TEST MOST LIKELY TO BE ABNORMAL IS:

A. Serum alkaline phosphatase
B. SGOT
C. SGPT
D. Ammonia tolerance test
E. Serum bilirubin

1166.   THE LEAST COMMON CLINICAL FINDING IS:

A. No signs or symptoms
B. Fever
C. Hypotension
D. Abdominal pain
E. Impending hepatic coma

1167.   THE MOST COMMON LABORATORY FINDING IS:

A. Ascitic leukocytosis
B. Peripheral blood leukopenia
C. Bacteria in stained ascitic fluid sediment
D. Positive blood culture
E. Normal peripheral white cell count

1168.   THE LEAST LIKELY POTENTIAL PATHOGENIC FACTOR WHICH
        MIGHT BE ENCOUNTERED IS:

A. Ascites
B. Esophageal varices
C. Jaundice
D. Prior paracentesis
E. An extra-abdominal focus of infection

Ref. Conn, H.O., Fessel, J.M.: Spontaneous Bacterial Peritonitis
in Cirrhosis: Variations on a Theme. Medicine, 50:161, 1971.

CASE HISTORY (QUESTIONS 1169-1170)

A 38 year-old trapper developed fever and painful swollen lymph nodes in the axilla 5 days after skinning about 500 muskrats. During the skinning, he sustained numerous minor cuts and abrasions on his hands. The next day he developed headache, anorexia, and several rigors. On examination: BP 120/70; P-118/min; T-40ºC (oral); R-20/min. He appeared acutely ill. A linear ulcer with thickened red margins was present on the left thumb. Several very tender large lymph nodes were palpable in the left axilla. A presumptive diagnosis of tularemia was made, and he received oral tetracycline 2 gm daily for 10 days. There was marked improvement. Eight days after completing the course of the tetracycline, fever recurred and tender lymph nodes recurred in the axilla. At this time agglutination tests for F. tularensis were positive (serum titer 1:400).

1169.   ANTIBIOTIC THERAPY FOR THE RECURRENCE SHOULD BE:
A.   Streptomycin
B.   Repeat tetracycline
C.   Gentamicin
D.   Chloramphenicol
E.   Sulfisoxazole

1170.   THE MOST COMMON CAUSE OF DEATH FROM TULAREMIA IS:
A.   Pneumonia   D.   Encephalitis
B.   Nephritis   E.   None of the above
C.   Shock
Ref. Walker, W. J., Moore, C. A.: Tularemia. CMA J, 105:390, 1971.

CASE HISTORY (QUESTIONS 1171-1175)

A 19 year-old Latin American woman suffered from chronic bilateral otitis media and sinusitis. 5 days previously a dental abscess had been drained. Progressive somnolence appeared with anorexia and a frontal headache. Because of an episide of unsteadiness and a possible seizure, she was brought to the hospital. On examination: BP 130/70; P-112/min; R-16/min; T-39.2ºC (rectal). There was a purulent nasal discharge. The site of the dental abscess appeared to be well healed. Both tympanic membranes were dull. There were no localizing neurologic signs. Peripheral WBC 18,000 (92% PMN). Spinal fluid examination 69 mg protein and 74 mg glucose/100 ml; 6 WBC; 0 RBC. Aerobic and anaerobic cultures were negative. EEG: slow waves over the right frontal area. Blood cultures negative. A diagnosis of brain abscess was made and therapy instituted.

1171.   IN REFERENCE TO THE MORTALITY RATE OF THIS DISEASE, WHICH IS CORRECT?:
A.   Overall mortality rate is 5%
B.   Intracerebral abscesses are more likely to cause death than subdural abscesses
C.   Overall mortality rate is about 40%
D.   Mortality rates have fallen from 40% to 20% in the last decade
E.   None of the above

1172.   THE CARDINAL SYMPTOM OF INTRACRANIAL INFECTION IS:
A.   Chills   D.   Headache
B.   Diplopia   E.   Confusion
C.   Tinnitus

1173. WHICH OF THE FOLLOWING IS MOST OFTEN ASSOCIATED WITH
INTRACRANIAL INFECTION?:
A. Fever
B. Localizing neurologic signs
C. Hypoglycorrhacia
D. Leukocytosis
E. Extracranial suppuration

1174. EVEN THOUGH A DEFINITIVE BACTERIOLOGIC DIAGNOSIS MAY
NOT BE AVAILABLE, THERAPY MUST BE INSTITUTED. THE BEST
ANTIBIOTIC TREATMENT FOR INITIAL THERAPY IS (PATIENT NOT
ALLERGIC TO PENICILLIN):
A. Erythromycin, by mouth, 250 mgm qid
B. Erythromycin as in A above, plus tetracycline by mouth 250 mgm qid
C. Penicillin, 20 million units daily, by intravenous route
D. Methicillin, 4 grams per day, by intravenous route
E. Penicillin, as in C above, plus chloramphenicol 2-4 gm per day by
intravenous route

1175. ADDITION OF CHLORAMPHENICOL TO THE REGIMEN, IF CHOSEN,
WOULD BE JUSTIFIED BECAUSE OF THE POSSIBLE PRESENCE OF
WHICH OF THE FOLLOWING?:
A. Bacteroides fragilis
B. Bacteroides oralis
C. Bacteroides melaninogenicus
D. Salmonella cholerasuis
E. Proteus vulgaris
Ref. Heinemann, H. S., Braude, A. I., Osterholm, J. L.: Intracranial
Suppurative Disease. JAMA, 218:1542, 1971.

CASE HISTORY (QUESTIONS 1176-1180)
A 20 year-old man presents to a hospital with headache, chills, and
fever. The physical examination is unremarkable except for a
fever of 41.3°C orally. He was discharged from the U. S. Army,
having served in Vietnam, 10 weeks prior to the current illness. On
questioning, he admitted to having neglected to complete his
chloroquine-primaquine chemoprophylaxis regimen.

1176. OF THE FOLLOWING DISEASES WHICH HE MAY HAVE ACQUIRED IN
VIETNAM, WHICH IS THE ONLY ONE WHICH COULD BE RESPONSIBLE
FOR HIS ILLNESS?:
A. Dengue fever
B. Scrub typhus
C. Malaria
D. Leptospirosis
E. Chikungunya virus infection

1177. A SMEAR OF BLOOD IS TAKEN AND MALARIA IS DIAGNOSED.
THE MOST LIKELY PARASITE IS:
A. P. vivax
B. P. falciparum
C. P. knowlesii
D. P. ovale

1178. OF THE FOLLOWING, THE MOST LIKELY PHYSICAL FINDING
WOULD BE:
A. Petechiae   D. Splenomegaly
B. Clubbing   E. Hemic murmur
C. Meningismus

1179.   WHICH OF THE FOLLOWING CHARACTERISTICS OF THE PARA-
        SITEMIA ARE <u>NOT</u> CHARACTERISTIC OF P. VIVAX INFECTION?:
        A.   Parasitized red cells are usually larger than non-parasitized cells
        B.   Schuffner's dots may be seen
        C.   Shizonts are seen in the blood
        D.   Mature gametocytes are "banana" shaped
        E.   Young ring forms occupy about 1/3 the diameter of the RBC

1180.   THE THERAPY FOR P. VIVAX INFECTIONS USES WHICH DRUGS?:
        A.   Chloroquine only
        B.   Chloroquine and primaquine
        C.   Quinine only
        D.   Pyrimethamine and sulfisoxazole
        E.   DDS
        Ref. Deller, J.J.: Malaria - Again a Diagnostic Consideration.
        A. F. P. , 5:68, 1972.

        CASE HISTORY (QUESTION 1181)
        A 16 year-old boy developed acute granulocytic leukemia. A remission
        was induced by the first chemotherapeutic regimen. Three months later
        relapse occurred, heralded by nausea, vomiting, and fever.
        On examination: T-41ºC (oral); BP 100/60; P-118; R22. Physical
        examination revealed only pallor and adynamic ileus. Blood cultures
        were obtained and therapy with polymyxin B was instituted. The blood
        cultures obtained on the third day of therapy contained <u>Aeromonas</u>
        hydrophilia.

1181.   TO WHICH OF THE FOLLOWING ANTIBIOTICS WOULD YOU EXPECT
        THIS ORGANISM TO BE SENSITIVE?:
        A.   Chloramphenicol and tetracycline
        B.   Colistin and polymyxin
        C.   Ampicillin
        D.   Penicillin
        Ref. Abrams, E. , Zierdt, C. H. , Brown, J. A.: Observations on
        Aeromonas Hydrophilia Septicemia in a Patient with Leukemia.
        <u>J Clin Path</u>, 24:491, 1971.

CASE HISTORY (QUESTIONS 1182-1185)

A 73 year-old woman was admitted for therapy of dehydration. She had been treated for 5 years with prednisone and chlorambucil for chronic lymphocytic leukemia. For 1 week prior to admission she had had dysuria and urinary frequency. Sixteen years ago she had carcinoma of the breast for which a radical mastectomy had been performed. On examination: T-37°C; P-88; R-18; BP 90/70. She was dehydrated and pale. No abnormal lymph nodes were felt. There were no nodules present along the mastectomy scar. The heart, lungs, abdomen and neurologic examination were normal. Laboratory date: Hct 29%; WBC 60,000/mm^3 (80% lymphocytes); BUN 42 mg; serum Cr 1.5 mg; Uric acid 7 mg; glucose 120 mg/100 ml; Chest X-ray normal. Urinalysis 50 WBC/hpf, numerous bacteria (culture 100,000 col E. coli/ml). In hospital she received intravenous fluids, prednisone, bufulsan and 1 gm of ampicillin orally per day. On the 6th day the temperature rose to 39°C. At that time the WBC was 16,000 (80% lymphocytes). Examination disclosed no findings except the following neurologic signs: weakness of abduction of the right eye and mild nuchal rigidity. A lumbar puncture was performed. The CSF was entirely normal. On the eighth hospital day sinus films revealed clouding of the sphenoid sinus. Examination now revelaed loss of abduction of both eyes, hoarse voice, bilateral ptosis, facial weakness, impaired swallowing, and inability to protrude the tongue. The temperature was 40°C. Another lumbar puncture showed cloudy fluid containing 250 white cells/mm^3 (85% polymorphonuclear cells, 15% monuclear cells), glucose 57 mg/100 ml (blood glucose 118 mg/ 100 ml). No bacteria were seen. The next day she became comatose. The CSF culture yielded P. aeruginosa. Shortly thereafter the patient died.

1182.   THE PHYSICAL EXAMINATION REVEALED DYSFUNCTION OF ALL THE FOLLOWING CRANIAL NERVES, EXCEPT:

A. III   D. X
B. VII   E. XII
C. V

1183.   THE INITIAL SPINAL FLUID CONTAINED NO WHITE CELLS, ALTHOUGH INFECTION OF THE CNS WITH P. AERUGINOSA LATER BECAME OBVIOUS. WHICH OF THE FOLLOWING SEEMS THE MOST LIKELY EXPLANATION?:

A. P. aeruginosa was not responsible for the CNS infection
B. Busulfan therapy
C. Prednisone therapy
D. Infection of meninges without communication to lower spinal space
E. None of the above

1184.   THE INITIAL CELLULAR RESPONSE (FIRST 1-2 DAYS) IN THE CSF DURING VIRAL MENINGITIS MAY BE POLYMORPHONUCLEAR. POLYMORPHONUCLEAR CELLS MAY CONSTITUTE WHAT FRACTION OF THE TOTAL CELL COUNT EARLY IN THE COURSE OF VIRAL MENINGITIS?:

A. 20
B. 35
C. 98
D. 50
E. 85

1185.   WHICH OF THE FOLLOWING ARGUES MOST STRONGLY AGAINST
         THIS COURSE BEING CAUSED BY A BRAIN ABSCESS?:
         A.   Negative blood cultures
         B.   Multiple cranial nerve palsies
         C.   Initially normal CSF analysis
         D.   No pulmonary focus
         E.   Only sphenoid sinus involved
         Ref. Case Records of the Massachusetts General Hospital Case 6-1972.
         New Eng J Med, 286:308, 1972.

         CASE HISTORY (QUESTION 1186)
         A 38 year-old R.N. punctured her hand with a needle contaminated with
         blood from a patient with post-transfusion hepatitis. Three months
         later she developed malaise, weakness, and lethargy. She
         recovered in two weeks at bed rest during which the peak SGOT reached
         2000 units/ml.

1186.   WHICH OF THE FOLLOWING STATEMENTS IS MOST LIKELY TO
         BE APPLICABLE TO THIS HISTORY?:
         A.   Patient has infectious hepatitis
         B.   Patient was infective for at least 1-2 weeks before she became ill
         C.   Patient is non-infectious for ward contacts
         D.   Testing patient for HAA prior to onset of symptoms would not
              have identified her as a risk to ward patients
         E.   None of the above
         Ref. Garibaldi, R.A., Rasmussen, C.N., Holmes, W.A., et al:
         Hospital Acquired Serum Hepatitis. JAMA, 219:1577, 1972.

         CASE HISTORY (QUESTION 1187)
         A 35 year-old man underwent resection of the superior segment of
         the right lower lobe for cavitary pulmonary tuberculosis. Post-
         operatively, he received INH for 2 years.

1187.   THE MOST EFFECTIVE WAY TO ESTIMATE THE ACTIVITY OF THIS
         MAN'S TUBERCULOSIS AT THE END OF THE TREATMENT
         PERIOD IS:
         A.   1st strength PPD
         B.   Laminograms of the right lower lobe
         C.   PA and lateral chest film
         D.   Sputum culture using 2% NaOH and acetylcysteine
         E.   None of the above
         Ref. Husen, L., Fulkerson, L.L., Del Vecchio, E., et al:
         Pulmonary Tuberculosis with Negative Findings on Chest X-Ray
         Films: A Study of 40 Cases. Chest, 60:540, 1971.

         CASE HISTORY (QUESTION 1188)
         A 29 year-old woman has been treated for 9 months with prednisone,
         6-mercaptopurine, and nitrogen mustard for acute leukemia. She
         developed fever, a severe headache, and a stiff neck. Gram's stain
         of the CSF revealed gram-positive rods, later identified as L.
         monocytogenes.

1188.   THE MOST EFFECTIVE ANTIBIOTIC REGIMEN WOULD BE
         TREATMENT WITH:
         A.   Chloramphenicol   D.   Gentamicin
         B.   Tetracycline   E.   Erythromycin
         C.   Penicillin and streptomycin
         Ref. Moellering, R.C., Medoff, G.C., Leech, I., et al: Antibiotic
         Synergism Against Listeria Monocytogenes. Antibicrob Ag Chemother,
         1:30, 1972.

CASE HISTORY (QUESTIONS 1189-1191)
A 29 year-old man underwent successful renal transplantation. On
the 19th postoperative day he became febrile. Four blood cultures
the next day contained Pseudomonas cepacia.

189.   THE TREATMENT OF CHOICE IS:
       A. Cephalothin
       B. Chloramphenicol
       C. Gentamicin
       D. Trimethoprim and sulphamethoxazole
       E. Polymyxin B.

190.   IN THE LABORATORY THE ORGANISM WOULD BE EXPECTED TO BE:
       A. Oxidase-positive
       B. Gram-negative
       C. Citrate-positive
       D. A glucose fermenter
       E. All of the above

1191. P. CEPACIA HAS BEEN ASSOCIATED WITH "FOOT ROT. " WHICH
       OF THE FOLLOWING ORGANISMS HAS BEEN THOUGHT TO PRO-
       DUCE A SIMILAR HYPERKERATOTIC, MACERATED, INFLAMMATORY
       FISSURING INFECTION OF THE FEET?:
       A. T. mentagrophytes   D. Corynebacterium sp.
       B. C. albicans   E. All of the above
       C. Staphylococci sp.
       Ref. Taplin, D. , Bassett, D. C. J. , Mertz, P. M. : Foot Lesions
       Associated with Pseudomonas Cepacia. Lancet, 2:568, 1971.

CASE HISTORY (QUESTIONS 1192-1193)
A 36 year-old woman under treatment for minimal active pulmonary
tuberculosis ingested a month's supply of INH, estimated to be about
10 grams, as a suicidal gesture. Two hours later she was examined
in an emergency room and appeared to be well. A few minutes later
she had a grand mal seizure, after which she was semi-comatose.

1192. INITIAL THERAPY SHOULD INCLUDE WHICH OF THE FOLLOWING?:
       A. Pyridoxine   D. Phenobarbital
       B. Streptomycin   E. None of the above
       C. Ammonium chloride

1193. OTHER MANIFESTATIONS OF INH POISONING INCLUDE ALL,
       EXCEPT:
       A. Albuminuria
       B. Hypotension
       C. Oliguria
       D. Severe metabolic alkalosis
       E. Cyanosis
       Ref. Brown, C. V. : Acute Isoniazid Poisoning. Amer Rev Resp Dis,
       105:206, 1972.

CASE HISTORY (QUESTIONS 1194-1196)
A 56 year-old man developed severe myalgia, headache, fever, and
an acute nonproductive cough. Within 24 hours he was prostrate but
alert. The cough persisted but there was no sputum production.
He had not been immunized against influenza, falling ill early in the
winter. On the third day of illness he became restless and complained
of shortness of breath. On examination he was agitated and there
was cyanosis of the lips; T-39.6°C; R-38; BP-110/84; P-128. The only
other abnormal findings were moist rales at the bases of both lungs.
WBC 7,600 (normal differential).

1194. WHICH OF THE FOLLOWING WOULD BEST REPRESENT THIS
       PATIENT'S ARTERIAL BLOOD GASES?:
       A. pH 6.9,pO_2 96,pCO_2 12
       B. pH 7.51,pO_2 41,pCO_2 19
       C. pH 7.45,pO_2 93,pCO_2 35
       D. pH 6.95,pO_2 35,pCO_2 65
       E. None of the above

1195. THE BEST METHOD FOR ADMINISTRATION OF OXYGEN TO THIS
       PATIENT WOULD BE:
       A. Oxygen not indicated - may terminate hypoxic respiratory drive
       B. Intranasal catheter
       C. Tank respiratory with room air
       D. Intermittent positive pressure with 100% oxygen
       E. 40% oxygen by face mask

1196. DESPITE INTENSIVE SUPPORTIVE TREATMENT THE PATIENT DIED.
       AT AUTOPSY THE HISTOPATHOLOGY WOULD MOST LIKELY SHOW?:
       A. Parenchymal polymorphonuclear infiltrate
       B. Microcolonies of bacteria
       C. Micro abscess in lung parenchyma
       D. Pulmonary capillary thrombi
       E. Interstitial edema
       Ref. Newton-John, H. F., Yung, A. P., Bennett, N. McK., et al:
       Influenza Virus Pneumonitis: A Report of Ten Cases. Med J Austral,
       2:1160, 1971.

CASE HISTORY (QUESTIONS 1197-1199)
A girl was born after a spontaneous premature labor at 33 weeks of
gestation. There had been no antenatal maternal illness. The
liquor was heavily stained with meconium. Becuase of respiratory
distress the baby was intubated and maintained on assisted respiration.
Two hours after birth the chest radiograph showed diffuse mottling and
peribronchial infiltration. Twelve hours after birth a generalized
macular and petechial erythema appeared. C. S. F. exam revealed
370 WBC/c. mm., protein 490 mg%; glucose 10 mg/ml. Gram-
positive bacilli were present in smears of the CSF and meconium.
Death occurred 38 hours after birth despite intravenous antibiotic
therapy and corticosteroids. L. monocytogenes was later cultured
from blood, CSF, and meconium.

1197. THE MOST COMMON FORM OF MATERNAL ILLNESS PRECEDING
       FATAL NEONATAL LISTERIOSIS IS:
       A. Influenza-like illness
       B. Septicemia
       C. Meningitis
       D. No specific illness
       E. Pneumonia

198.   AT AUTOPSY, THE LUNGS WOULD MOST LIKELY SHOW:
        A. Bland infarcts
        B. Interstitial lymphocytic infiltrate
        C. Neutrophilic exudate in alveolar ducts and bronchioles
        D. Hyaline membrane
        E. None of the above

199.   THE ANTIBIOTIC PREFERRED FOR TREATMENT OF NEONATAL
        LISTERIOSIS IS:
        A. Tetracycline   D. Penicillin
        B. Chloramphenicol   E. Ampicillin
        C. Oxytetracycline
        Ref. Bush, R. T.: Purulent Meningitis of the Newborn: A Survey of
        28 Cases. New Zealand Med J, 73:278, 1971.

        CASE HISTORY (QUESTIONS 1200-1201)
        A 52 year-old woman was admitted to hospital for high fever,
        headache, and weakness. T-102.5°F; P-108/min; R-20/min;
        BP-90/50. No localizing physical findings were observed. WBC
        28,000/cu mm. Ampicillin was administered after a single blood
        culture was obtained. For 4-6 hours after 4 gm of ampicillin had
        been given intravenously, 3 more blood cultures were obtained. The
        initial blood culture contained K. pneumoniae. The subsequent
        3 blood cultures were cloudy and contained a gram-negative filament
        20-100 microns long.

1200.   THESE FINDINGS MOST LIKELY REPRESENT:
        A. Polymicrobic gram-negative sepsis
        B. An artifact
        C. Aberrant form of K. pneumoniae
        D. Presence of Vibrio fetus in blood
        E. None of the above

1201.   FURTHER EXAMINATIONS OF THE BLOOD CULTURES WHICH CONTAIN
        FILAMENTOUS FORMS SHOULD INCLUDE:
        A. Subculture in the presence of ampicillin
        B. Anaerobic culture
        C. Serotyping of filamentous forms with K. pneumoniae antisera
        D. Wright's stain
        E. Acid fast stain
        Ref. Lorian, V., Waluschka, A.: Blood Cultures Showing Aberrant
        Forms of Bacteria. Amer J Clin Path, 57:406, 1972.

CASE HISTORY (QUESTIONS 1202-1203)
A 39 year-old man sustained 3rd degree burns over 65% of the body surfa
In the hospital he received appropriate intravenous fluids. The burns
were covered with mafenide acetate. He also received 600,000 units
of aqueous penicillin every 6 hours through an indwelling central
venous line. Perineal burns necessitated urinary drainage through a
closed system, irrigated with neomycin-polymyxin solution four times
per day. On the 12th hospital day cultures of the burns from several
areas show pure cultures of a yeast.

1202.   WHICH OF THE FOLLOWING WOULD BE MOST HELPFUL IN
        DISTINGUISHING COLONIZATION FROM INFECTION?:
        A.   Speciation of the yeast
        B.   A blood culture
        C.   A urine culture
        D.   Grocott-stained, full-thickness biopsy of wound
        E.   Repeat wound culture

1203.   WHICH OF THE FOLLOWING ARE APPROPRIATE MANEUVERS
        UNDER THESE CIRCUMSTANCES?:
        A.   Discontinue mafenide acetate
        B.   Stop penicillin
        C.   Remove CVP line
        D.   All of the above
        E.   B and C only
        Ref. MacMillan, B.G., Law, E.J., Holder, I.A.: Experience
        with Candida Infections in the Burn Patient. Arch Surg, 104:509, 1972.

FOUR OF THE FIVE SITUATIONS IN THE NUMBERED LIST BELOW
ARE COMMON TO ONE OF THE THREE FUNCTIONAL DISTURBANCES
DESIGNATED BY LETTER. SELECT THE ONE NUMBERED
SITUATION WHICH IS THE EXCEPTION AND THE LETTERED
FUNCTIONAL DISTURBANCE COMMON TO THE REMAINING FOUR
NUMBERED SITUATIONS:

SITUATION	FUNCTIONAL DISTURBANCE
1. Tuberculosis	A. Pleural effusion with high
2. Bronchogenic carcinoma	protein content
3. Metastatic tumor	B. Empyema
4. Pulmonary infarction	C. Pleural effusion with low
5. Sarcoid	protein content

1204. Situation
1205. Functional disturbance
Ref. Ball, W. C., Jr.: Pleural Effusions, Chap 41 in The Principles
and Practice of Medicine, 17th Ed., Appleton-Century-Crofts,
New York, 1968, pp. 410-415.

SITUATION	FUNCTIONAL DISTURBANCE
1. Spirillum minus infection	A. Relapsing or recurrent fever
2. Borellia infection	B. Sustained fever
3. Chronic meningococcemia	C. Hectic fever
4. Psittacosis	
5. Brucellosis	

1206. Situation
1207. Functional disturbance
Ref. Fekety, F. R., Cluff, L. E.: The Clinical and Laboratory
Manifestations of Infectious Diseases in The Principles and Practice
of Medicine, 17th Ed., Appleton-Century-Crofts, New York, 1968,
pp. 654-671.

SITUATION	FUNCTIONAL DISTURBANCE
1. Typhoid fever	A. Sinus tachycardia
2. Tularemia	B. Atrial flutter
3. Psittacosis	C. Sinus bradycardia
4. Central nervous system infection	
5. Influenza	

1208. Situation
1209. Functional disturbance
Ref. Fekety, F. R., Cluff, L. E.: The Clinical and Laboratory
Manifestations of Infectious Diseases in The Principles and Practice
of Internal Medicine, 17th Ed., Chap 66, Appleton-Century-Crofts,
New York, 1968, pp. 654-671.

SITUATION	FUNCTIONAL DISTURBANCE
1. Tuberculosis	A. Eosinophilia
2. Scarlet fever	B. Monocytosis
3. Histoplasmosis	C. Megakaryocytosis
4. Rocky Mountain Spotted Fever	
5. Influenza	

1210.   Situation
1211.   Functional disturbance
Ref. Fekety, F. R. , Cluff, L. E.: The Clinical and Laboratory
Manifestations of Infectious Diseases in The Principles and Practice
of Internal Medicine, 17th Ed. , Chap 66, Appleton-Centruy-Crofts,
New York, 1968, pp. 654-671.

SITUATION	FUNCTIONAL DISTURBANCE
1. Clostridium welchii infection	A. Diarrhea, tenesmus, fever
2. Amebic dysentery	B. No diarrhea, vomiting, fever
3. Giardia lamblia infection	C. Diarrhea, tenesmus, little
4. ECHO virus infection	or no fever
5. Coxsackie virus infection	

1212.   Situation
1213.   Functional disturbance
Ref. Fekety, F. R.: Cluff, L. E.: The Clinical and Laboratory
Manifestations of Infectious Diseases in The Principles and Practice
of Medicine, 17th Ed. , Chap 66, Appleton-Century-Crofts, New York,
1968, pp. 654-671.

SITUATION	FUNCTIONAL DISTURBANCE
1. Influenza virus infection	A. Laryngitis in children
2. Adenovirus infection	B. Croup in children
3. Respiratory syncytial virus infection	C. Pleurodynia
4. Parainfluenza virus infection	
5. Rhinovirus infection	

1214.   Situation
1215.   Functional disturbance
Ref. Fekety, F. R.: Influenza and Other Viral Respiratory Diseases in
The Principles and Practice of Medicine, 17th Ed. , Chap 72,
Appleton-Century-Crofts, New York, 1968, pp. 718-723.

SITUATION	FUNCTIONAL DISTURBANCE
1. Erythema multiforme	A. Leukopenia
2. Scarlet fever	B. Mastocytosis
3. Diphtheria	C. Eosinophilia
4. Hookworm infestation	
5. Antibiotic sensitivity	

1216.   Situation
1217.   Functional disturbance
Ref. Owen, A. H. , Jr.: Disorders of White Cells: General Considerations in The Principles and Practice of Medicine, 17th Ed. , Chap 57,
Appleton-Century-Crofts, New York, 1968, pp. 558-565.

SITUATION	FUNCTIONAL DISTURBANCE
1. Brucellosis	A. Plasmacytosis
2. Subacute bacterial endocarditis	B. Monocytosis
3. Rocky Mountain spotted fever	C. Macrocytosis
4. Tuberculosis	
5. Scarlet fever	

1218. Situation
1219. Functional disturbance
Ref. Owen, A. H., Jr.: Disorders of White Cells: General Considerations in The Principles and Practice of Medicine, 17th Ed., Chap 57, Appleton-Century-Crofts, New York, 1968, pp. 558-565.

SITUATION	FUNCTIONAL DISTURBANCE
1. Q fever pneumonia	A. Scant sputum
2. Adenovirus pneumonia	B. Erythema nodosum
3. Gr A beta hemolytic streptococcal pneumonia	C. Multiple chills
4. Measles pneumonia	
5. Varicella pneumonia	

1220. Situation
1221. Functional disturbance
Ref. Carpenter, C. J., Jr., Mulholland, J. H.: Pneumonia in The Principles and Practice of Medicine, 17th Ed., Chap 73, Appleton-Century-Crofts, New York, 1968, pp. 723-736.

SITUATION	FUNCTIONAL DISTURBANCE
1. Hodgkin's disease	A. Salmonella septicemia
2. Sickle cell disease	B. Leukopenia
3. Malaria	C. Arthralgia
4. Bartonellosis	
5. Rheumatic fever	

1222. Situation
1223. Functional disturbance
Ref. Wolfe, M. S., Armstrong, D., Louria, D. B., et al: Salmonellosis in Patients with Neoplastic Diseases. Arch Intern Med, 128:546, 1971.

SITUATION	FUNCTIONAL DISTURBANCE
1. Reticular dysgenesis	A. Impaired immunoglobulin production
2. Ataxia telangectasia	
3. Wiskott-Aldrich syndrome	B. Deficient phagocytosis
4. Chronic granulomatous disease	C. Immunoglobulin deficiency combined with impaired cellular hypersensitivity
5. Swiss type hypogammaglobulinemia	

1224. Situation
1225. Functional disturbance
Ref. Allen, J. C.: Recurrent Infections in Man Associated with Immunologic or Phagocytic Deficiencies. Postgrad Med, 50:88, 1971.

SITUATION	FUNCTIONAL DISTURBANCE
1. Infectious mononucleosis	A. Lymphocytosis
2. Burkitt's lymphoma	B. Antibody to Epstein-Barr
3. Systemic lupus erythematosus	virus
4. Nasopharyngeal carcinoma	C. Renal insufficiency
5. G-6 PD deficiency	

1226. Situation
1227. Functional disturbance
Ref. Evan, A. S.: The Spectrum of Infections with Epstein-Barr Virus:
A Hypothesis. J Inf Dis, 124:330, 1971.

SITUATION	FUNCTIONAL DISTURBANCE
1. Asymptomatic infection	A. Antibody to Epstein-Barr
2. Tonsillitis without lymphadenopathy	virus after infection
3. Infectious mononucleosis	B. Isolation of cytomegalovirus
4. Cytomegalovirus infection	C. Anemia
5. Non-cytomegalovirus transfusion	
mononucleosis	

1228. Situation
1229. Functional disturbance
Ref. Evans, A. S.: The Spectrum of Infection with Epstein-Barr Virus:
A Hypothesis. J Inf Dis, 124:330, 1971.

SITUATION	FUNCTIONAL DISTURBANCE
1. Convulsions	A. Pneumothorax
2. Tachypnea	B. Intracranial hemorrhage
3. Abdominal distention	C. Neonatal bacterial sepsis
4. Jaundice	
5. Intracranial calcifications	

1230. Situation
1231. Functional disturbance
Ref. Gotoff, S., Behrman, R. E.: Neonatal Septicemia. J Ped,
76:142, 1970.

SITUATION	FUNCTIONAL DISTURBANCE
1. Fever	A. Tuberculous peritonitis
2. Abdominal pain	B. Pancreatitis
3. Abnormal X-ray of chest	C. Spontaneous peritonitis
4. Polymorphonuclear ascitic	
leukocytosis	
5. Serum hyperbilirubinemia	

1232. Situation
1233. Functional disturbance
Ref. Conn, H. O., Fessel, J. M.: Spontaneous Bacterial Peritonitis in
Cirrhosis: Variations on a Theme. Medicine, 50:161, 1971.

SITUATION	FUNCTIONAL DISTURBANCE
1. Measles	A. Vesicles
2. Smallpox	B. Pustules
3. Chickenpox	C. Positive Weil-Felix test
4. Rickettsialpox	
5. Dermatitis venenata	

234.   Situation
235.   Functional disturbance
Ref. Leg, H. L.: Rickettsialpox. Textbook of Medicine, 13th Ed.,
Beeson, P. B., McDermott, W., (Ed), W. B. Saunders Co., Philadelphia,
1971, p. 482.

SITUATION	FUNCTIONAL DISTURBANCE
1. Bephenium therapy	A. Retinal damage
2. Amodiaquine therapy	B. Cardiac arrhythmia
3. Emetene therapy	C. Nausea, vomiting
4. Paromomycin therapy	
5. Thiabendazole therapy	

1236.   Situation
1237.   Functional therapy
Ref. Clinical Parasitology, Faust, E. C., Russell, P. F., Jung, R. C.,
(Ed), 8th Edition, Lea and Febiger, Philadelphia, 1970, p. 166, 219,
315, 326.

SITUATION	FUNCTIONAL DISTURBANCE
1. Rheumatic fever	A. Pleural effusion occurs
2. Pancreatitis	frequently
3. Systemic lupus erythematous	B. Rarely accompanied by
4. Coxsackie B pneumonia	pleural fluid
5. Pleural mesothelioma	C. Pericarditis usually seen

1238.   Situation
1239.   Functional disturbance
Ref. Ball, W. C., Jr.: Pleural Effusions, Chap 41 in The Principles
and Practice of Medicine, 17th Ed., Appleton-Century-Crofts,
New York, 1968, pp. 410-415.

SITUATION	FUNCTIONAL DISTURBANCE
1. Pain in hip	A. Retroperitoneal abscess
2. Fever	B. Septic arthritis of hip
3. Limp	C. Urinary tract infection
4. Tenderness of thigh	
5. Rectal mass or tenderness	

1240.   Situation
1241.   Functional disturbance
Ref. March, A. W., Riley, L. H., Robinson, R. A.: Retroperitoneal
Abscess and Septic Arthritis of the Hip in Children. J Bone Joint Surg,
54A: 67, 1972.

The author has made every effort to thoroughly verify the questions and answers; however, in a volume of this size, some ambiguities and possible inaccuracies may appear. Therefore, if in doubt, consult your references.

THE PUBLISHERS

SECTION I

1. B	48. D	95. C	142. C	189. D
2. E	49. D	96. B	143. B	190. D
3. D	50. D	97. A	144. C	191. C
4. E	51. E	98. A	145. B	192. C
5. A	52. A	99. B	146. C	193. A
6. B	53. E	100. A	147. B	194. A
7. E	54. E	101. A	148. A	195. B
8. D	55. D	102. C	149. C	196. C
9. D	56. E	103. A	150. A	197. A
10. D	57. A	104. A	151. B	198. E
11. E	58. B	105. A	152. B	199. A
12. A	59. A	106. B	153. C	200. E
13. C	60. C	107. A	154. D	201. E
14. B	61. E	108. A	155. A	202. A
15. B	62. A	109. C	156. B	203. E
16. E	63. A	110. C	157. D	204. D
17. C	64. A	111. A	158. B	205. B
18. C	65. C	112. C	159. B	206. E
19. B	66. A	113. D	160. A	207. A
20. D	67. E	114. D	161. D	208. A
21. E	68. A	115. D	162. C	209. A
22. E	69. C	116. C	163. A	210. A
23. B	70. A	117. A	164. B	211. E
24. D	71. C	118. C	165. C	212. E
25. D	72. A	119. D	166. C	213. E
26. A	73. E	120. C	167. C	214. E
27. D	74. A	121. C	168. D	215. A
28. B	75. A	122. C	169. C	216. E
29. A	76. B	123. C	170. C	217. A
30. D	77. C	124. B	171. D	218. E
31. A	78. B	125. C	172. D	219. E
32. C	79. B	126. C	173. A	220. E
33. D	80. C	127. C	174. A	221. E
34. B	81. B	128. C	175. B	222. E
35. D	82. B	129. C	176. A	223. E
36. D	83. B	130. C	177. B	224. A
37. E	84. B	131. C	178. A	225. E
38. B	85. A	132. A	179. D	226. B
39. A	86. C	133. B	180. A	227. C
40. E	87. A	134. B	181. B	228. E
41. A	88. A	135. C	182. D	229. A
42. C	89. A	136. B	183. C	230. A
43. C	90. B	137. C	184. C	231. B
44. B	91. C	138. D	185. C	232. C
45. A	92. A	139. D	186. B	233. D
46. D	93. B	140. A	187. C	234. A
47. B	94. B	141. C	188. D	235. E

236. E	291. A	343. A	398. A	453. C
237. D	292. C	344. C	399. B	454. C
238. E	293. D	345. A	400. B	455. B
239. A	294. A	346. A	401. A	456. A
240. B	295. A	347. E	402. C	457. C
241. C	296. B	348. A	403. D	458. B
242. D	297. B	349. A	404. A	459. A
243. D	298. C	350. A	405. D	460. D
244. F	299. B	351. C	406. B	461. C
245. E	300. D	352. B	407. C	462. C
246. B	301. B	353. A	408. B	463. A
247. A	302. A	354. C	409. C	464. B
248. C	303. C	355. B	410. B	465. B
249. B	304. D	356. B	411. B	466. A
250. A	305. D	357. A	412. B	467. D
251. C	306. D	358. C	413. C	468. C
252. D	307. B	359. A	414. C	469. B
253. A	308. C	360. B	415. B	470. A
254. F	309. A	361. A	416. C	471. D
255. E	310. E	362. B	417. B	472. C
256. E	311. D	363. C	418. D	473. E
257. D	312. B	364. A	419. C	474. D
258. G	313. C	365. B	420. B	475. A
259. A	314. A	366. B	421. A	476. C
260. B	315. E	367. C	422. B	477. B
261. D	316. D	368. C	423. C	478. C
262. F	317. A	369. C	424. B	479. A
263. E	318. E	370. C	425. C	480. D
264. C	319. F	371. D	426. A	481. E
265. B	320. D	372. C	427. D	482. B
266. D	321. C	373. A	428. A	483. B
267. A	322. B	374. B	429. E	484. A
268. C		375. A	430. C	485. D
269. B	SECTION II	376. B	431. C	486. C
270. C		377. A	432. C	487. A
271. C	323. A	378. B	433. E	488. C
272. B	324. E	379. D	434. C	489. B
273. A	325. D	380. A	435. A	490. A
274. A	326. E	381. B	436. B	491. E
275. E	327. E	382. A	437. E	492. C
276. C	328. C	383. C	438. E	493. D
277. D	329. D	384. C	439. D	494. E, B
278. B	330. A	385. D	440. C	495. F
279. B	331. B	386. A	441. B	496. C
280. A	332. B	387. C	442. B	497. D
281. C	333. E	388. A	443. E	498. A
282. D	334. A	389. B	444. A	
283. F	335. A	390. C	445. B	SECTION III
284. E	336. A	391. C	446. C	
285. C	337. A	392. C	447. D	499. E
286. C	338. B	393. D	448. E	500. E
287. B	339. B	394. C	449. B	501. E
288. A	340. E	395. B	450. A	502. C
289. C	341. A	396. D	451. B	503. D
290. B	342. A	397. C	452. C	504. C

505.	E	560.	B	615.	A	667.	D	722.	A
506.	C	561.	D	616.	C	668.	B	723.	C
507.	E	562.	D	617.	B	669.	B	724.	E
508.	E	563.	A	618.	D	670.	E	725.	A
509.	A	564.	B	619.	E	671.	C	726.	C
510.	B	565.	B	620.	B	672.	C	727.	C
511.	C	566.	A	621.	C	673.	A	728.	A
512.	E	567.	D	622.	A	674.	A	729.	A
513.	A	568.	A	623.	D	675.	C	730.	A
514.	E	569.	B			676.	B	731.	B
515.	C	570.	C	**SECTION IV**		677.	A	732.	B
516.	C	571.	C			678.	A	733.	C
517.	D	572.	C	624.	C	679.	A	734.	C
518.	E	573.	C	625.	D	680.	A	735.	B
519.	E	574.	C	626.	C	681.	A	736.	A
520.	D	575.	C	627.	E	682.	B	737.	B
521.	C	576.	C	628.	E	683.	A	738.	C
522.	E	577.	C	629.	A	684.	B	739.	C
523.	C	578.	B	630.	C	685.	B	740.	C
524.	A	579.	C	631.	D	686.	B	741.	B
525.	B	580.	B	632.	C	687.	C	742.	C
526.	C	581.	A	633.	C	688.	C	743.	B
527.	A	582.	B	634.	D	689.	A	744.	B
528.	A	583.	B	635.	E	690.	C	745.	B
529.	A	584.	A	636.	E	691.	B	746.	B
530.	C	585.	D	637.	B	692.	C	747.	A
531.	A	586.	E	638.	B	693.	E	748.	B
532.	A	587.	D	639.	E	694.	A	749.	B
533.	A	588.	A	640.	E	695.	D	750.	B
534.	A	589.	E	641.	D	696.	C	751.	B
535.	D	590.	D	642.	A	697.	B	752.	B
536.	A	591.	D	643.	E	698.	A	753.	C
537.	C	592.	E	644.	E	699.	B	754.	A
538.	B	593.	B	645.	C	700.	A	755.	C
539.	B	594.	E	646.	D	701.	B	756.	B
540.	A	595.	B	647.	B	702.	A	757.	B
541.	B	596.	E	648.	B	703.	D	758.	C
542.	B	597.	E	649.	D	704.	C	759.	C
543.	C	598.	C	650.	B	705.	A	760.	A
544.	C	599.	E	651.	D	706.	C	761.	A
545.	B	600.	B	652.	C	707.	A	762.	C
546.	B	601.	C	653.	C	708.	A	763.	C
547.	B	602.	A	654.	E	709.	D	764.	C
548.	B	603.	A	655.	D	710.	E	765.	A
549.	B	604.	E	656.	D	711.	A	766.	B
550.	A	605.	A	657.	D	712.	A	767.	B
551.	C	606.	C	658.	E	713.	A	768.	A
552.	B	607.	B	659.	B	714.	B	769.	A
553.	A	608.	A	660.	E	715.	E	770.	C
554.	B	609.	A	661.	A	716.	C	771.	C
555.	A	610.	D	662.	B	717.	D	772.	B
556.	B	611.	A	663.	E	718.	E	773.	C
557.	D	612.	C	664.	E	719.	A	774.	A
558.	A	613.	B	665.	C	720.	C	775.	A
559.	B	614.	B	666.	C	721.	B	776.	B

777.	B	832.	E	887.	D	939.	A	991.	B
778.	B	833.	E	888.	B	940.	B	992.	B
779.	B	834.	A	889.	C	941.	C, D	993.	A
780.	C	835.	C	890.	A	942.	B	994.	A
781.	B	836.	A	891.	A	943.	B	995.	A
782.	B	837.	E	892.	C	944.	A	996.	A
783.	A	838.	B	893.	B	945.	D	997.	E
784.	B	839.	E	894.	A	946.	C	998.	A
785.	D	840.	A	895.	D	947.	E	999.	B
786.	D	841.	C	896.	C	948.	G	1000.	C
787.	B	842.	F	897.	E	949.	F	1001.	A
788.	A	843.	G	898.	B	950.	C	1002.	B
789.	C	844.	D	899.	E	951.	A	1003.	B
790.	C	845.	C	900.	A	952.	B	1004.	C
791.	A	846.	A	901.	D	953.	D	1005.	B
792.	B	847.	B	902.	C	954.	A	1006.	C
793.	B	848.	A	903.	B	955.	A	1007.	C
794.	B	849.	D	904.	E	956.	C	1008.	C
795.	D	850.	F	905.	D	957.	B	1009.	C
796.	B	851.	A	906.	B	958.	A	1010.	A
797.	A	852.	G	907.	C	959.	D	1011.	C
798.	A	853.	F	908.	A	960.	A	1012.	D
799.	D	854.	E			961.	B	1013.	B
800.	B	855.	G	SECTION V		962.	E	1014.	A
801.	A	856.	E			963.	A	1015.	D
802.	C	857.	D	909.	C	964.	D	1016.	D
803.	C	858.	C	910.	C	965.	C	1017.	B
804.	B	859.	F	911.	D	966.	C	1018.	C
805.	C	860.	G	912.	C			1019.	B
806.	C	861.	C	913.	B	SECTION VI		1020.	A
807.	D	862.	D	914.	A			1021.	B
808.	D	863.	B	915.	B	967.	A	1022.	A
809.	C	864.	E	916.	B	968.	E	1023.	A
810.	D	865.	A	917.	C	969.	A	1024.	B
811.	D	866.	A	918.	A	970.	C	1025.	D
812.	D	867.	A	919.	A	971.	D	1026.	B
813.	B	868.	C	920.	A	972.	B	1027.	E
814.	C	869.	B	921.	A	973.	C	1028.	C
815.	E	870.	A	922.	A	974.	E	1029.	B
816.	B	871.	A	923.	B	975.	D	1030.	A
817.	C	872.	B	924.	C	976.	A	1031.	A
818.	E	873.	C	925.	D	977.	C	1032.	E
819.	C	874.	B	926.	A	978.	C	1033.	C
820.	A	875.	A	927.	A	979.	B	1034.	A
821.	C	876.	B	928.	C	980.	A	1035.	C
822.	D	877.	B	929.	A	981.	D	1036.	E
823.	E	878.	A	930.	E	982.	B	1037.	A
824.	D	879.	C	931.	B	983.	D	1038.	A
825.	A	880.	A	932.	C	984.	C	1039.	D
826.	A	881.	B	933.	B	985.	B	1040.	E
827.	C	882.	D	934.	A	986.	C	1041.	E
828.	E	883.	B	935.	E	987.	A	1042.	E
829.	C	884.	A	936.	A	988.	A	1043.	B
830.	E	885.	C	937.	A	989.	A	1044.	E
831.	A	886.	D	938.	B	990.	B	1045.	B

1046.	A	1098.	E	1153.	C	1205.	A
1047.	B	1099.	E	1154.	B	1206.	4
1048.	E	1100.	E	1155.	E	1207.	A
1049.	B	1101.	E	1156.	C	1208.	5
1050.	B	1102.	B	1157.	A	1209.	C
1051.	A	1103.	E	1158.	B	1210.	2
1052.	A	1104.	D	1159.	C	1211.	B
1053.	C	1105.	B	1160.	E	1212.	2
1054.	A	1106.	C	1161.	C	1213.	C
1055.	A	1107.	D	1162.	B	1214.	2
1056.	B	1108.	A	1163.	A	1215.	A
1057.	A	1109.	A	1164.	B	1216.	3
1058.	C	1110.	C	1165.	E	1217.	C
1059.	D	1111.	E	1166.	C	1218.	5
1060.	D	1112.	E	1167.	A	1219.	B
1061.	A	1113.	C	1168.	E	1220.	3
1062.	B	1114.	B	1169.	B	1221.	A
1063.	C	1115.	D	1170.	A	1222.	5
1064.	E	1116.	A	1171.	C	1223.	A
1065.	E	1117.	C	1172.	D	1224.	4
1066.	C	1118.	D	1173.	E	1225.	A
1067.	D	1119.	E	1174.	E	1226.	5
1068.	B	1120.	A	1175.	A	1227.	B
1069.	B	1121.	E	1176.	C	1228.	4
		1122.	C	1177.	A	1229.	A
SECTION VII		1123.	B	1178.	D	1230.	5
		1124.	C	1179.	D	1231.	C
1070.	C	1125.	E	1180.	B	1232.	3
1071.	B	1126.	D	1181.	A	1233.	C
1072.	D	1127.	A	1182.	C	1234.	2
1073.	E	1128.	A	1183.	D	1235.	A
1074.	B	1129.	C	1184.	E	1236.	3
1075.	B	1130.	B	1185.	B	1237.	C
1076.	A	1131.	E	1186.	B	1238.	4
1077.	E	1132.	C	1187.	D	1239.	A
1078.	C	1133.	B	1188.	C	1240.	5
1079.	E	1134.	C	1189.	D	1241.	B
1080.	C	1135.	D	1190.	E		
1081.	E	1136.	E	1191.	E		
1082.	C	1137.	B	1192.	A		
1083.	C	1138.	A	1193.	D		
1084.	B	1139.	B	1194.	B		
1085.	E	1140.	B	1195.	D		
1086.	A	1141.	D	1196.	E		
1087.	B	1142.	C	1197.	D		
1088.	C	1143.	A	1198.	C		
1089.	B	1144.	D	1199.	E		
1090.	B	1145.	C	1200.	C		
1091.	C	1146.	C	1201.	D		
1092.	D	1147.	D	1202.	D		
1093.	A	1148.	C	1203.	D		
1094.	D	1149.	B				
1095.	B	1150.	B	**SECTION VIII**			
1096.	A	1151.	A				
1097.	C	1152.	E	1204.	5		

sem

**AVAILABLE AT YOUR LOCAL BOOKSTORE
OR USE THIS ORDER FORM**

MEDICAL EXAMINATION PUBLISHING CO., INC.

65-36 Fresh Meadow Lane, Flushing, N.Y. 11365

Date: _____

Please send me the following books:

_____

_____

_____

_____

_____

☐ Payment enclosed to save postage.

☐ Bill me. I will remit payment within 30 days.

Name _____

Address _____

City & State _____ Zip _____

(Please print)

OTHER BOOKS AVAILABLE

Quan.	I T E M S	Code	Unit Price	Quan.	I T E M S	Code	Unit Price
	MEDICAL EXAM REVIEW BOOKS				**SPEC. BOARD REV. BKS.** *(Cont'd.)*		
	Vol. 1 Comprehensive	101	$12.00		Family Practice Specialty Board Review	309	$10.00
	Vol. 2 Clinical Medicine	102	7.00		Internal Medicine Specialty Board Review	303	10.00
	Vol. 2A Txtbk. Study Guide of Int. Med.	123	7.00		Neurology Specialty Board Review	306	10.00
	Vol. 2B Txtbk. Study Guide of Int. Med.	130	7.00		Obstetrics-Gynecology Spec. Bd. Review	304	10.00
	Vol. 3 Basic Sciences	103	7.00		Pathology Specialty Board Review	305	10.00
	Vol. 4 Obstetrics-Gynecology	104	7.00		Pediatrics Specialty Board Review	301	10.00
	Vol. 4A Textbk. Study Guide of Gynecology	152	7.00		Physical Medicine Spec. Bd. Review	308	10.00
	Vol. 5 Surgery	105	7.00		Surgery Specialty Board Review	302	10.00
	Vol. 5A Textbk. Study Guide of Surgery	150	7.00		The Psychiatry Boards	307	8.00
	Vol. 6 Public Health & Prev. Medicine	106	7.00		**STATE BOARD REVIEW BOOKS**		
	Vol. 8 Psychiatry & Neurology	108	7.00		Medical State Board Exam. Rev. - Part 1	411	9.00
	Vol.11 Pediatrics	111	7.00		Medical State Board Exam. Rev. - Part 2	412	9.00
	Vol.12 Anesthesiology	112	7.00		Cardiopulmonary Techn. Exam. Rev.-Vol.1	473	7.00
	Vol.13 Orthopaedics	113	10.00		Dental Exam. Review Book - Vol. 1	431	7.50
	Vol.14 Urology	114	10.00		Dental Exam. Review Book - Vol. 2	432	7.50
	Vol.15 Ophthalmology	115	10.00		Dental Exam. Review Book - Vol. 3	433	7.50
	Vol.16 Otolaryngology	116	10.00		Dental Hygiene Exam. Review - Vol. 1	461	7.00
	Vol.17 Radiology	117	10.00		Emergency Med. Techn. Exam. Rev. - Vol.1	465	7.00
	Vol.18 Thoracic Surgery	118	10.00		Emergency Med. Techn. Exam. Rev. - Vol.2	466	7.00
	Vol.19 Neurological Surgery	119	15.00		Immunology Exam. Review Book - Vol. 1	424	7.00
	Vol.20 Physical Medicine	128	10.00		Inhalation Therapy Exam. Review - Vol. 1	471	7.00
	Vol.21 Dermatology	127	10.00		Inhalation Therapy Exam. Review - Vol. 2	344	7.00
	Vol.22 Gastroenterology	141	10.00		Laboratory Asst. Exam. Rev. Bk. - Vol. 1	455	7.00
	Vol.23 Child Psychiatry	126	10.00		Medical Librarian Exam. Rev. Bk. - Vol. 1	495	7.00
	Vol.24 Pulmonary Diseases	143	10.00		Medical Record Library Science - Vol. 1	496	7.00
	ECFMG Exam Review - Part One	120	7.00		Medical Techn. Exam. Review - Vol. 1	451	7.00
	ECFMG Exam Review - Part Two	121	7.00		Medical Techn. Exam. Review - Vol. 2	452	7.00
	BASIC SCIENCE REVIEW BOOKS				Occupational Therapy Exam. Rev. - Vol.1	475	7.00
	Anatomy Review	201	6.00		Pharmacy Exam. Review Book - Vol. 1	421	7.00
	Biochemistry Review	202	6.00		Physical Therapy Exam. Review - Vol. 1	481	7.00
	Heart & Vascular Systems Basic Sciences	212	7.00		Physical Therapy Exam. Review - Vol. 2	482	7.00
	Microbiology Review	203	6.00		X-Ray Technology Exam. Rev. - Vol. 1	441	7.00
	Nervous System Basic Sciences	210	7.00		X-Ray Technology Exam. Rev. - Vol. 2	442	7.00
	Pathology Review	204	6.00		**NURSING EXAM REVIEW BOOKS**		
	Pharmacology Review	205	6.00		Vol. 1 Medical-Surgical Nursing	501	4.00
	Physiology Review	206	6.00		Vol. 2 Psychiatric-Mental Health Nursing	502	4.00
	Respiratory System Basic Sciences	213	7.00		Vol. 3 Maternal-Child Health Nursing	503	4.00
	Anatomy Textbook Study Guide	124	7.00		Vol. 4 Basic Sciences	504	4.00
	Histology Textbook Study Guide	151	7.00		Vol. 5 Anatomy and Physiology	505	4.00
	Medical Physiology Textbk. Study Guide	155	7.00		Vol. 6 Pharmacology	506	4.00
	SPECIALTY BOARD REVIEW BOOKS				Vol. 7 Microbiology	507	4.00
	Dermatology Specialty Board Review	311	10.00		*(Continued on reverse side)*		

Prices subject to change

OTHER BOOKS AVAILABLE

Quan.	I T E M S	Code	Unit Price	Quan.	I T E M S	Code	Unit Price
	Vol. 8 Nutrition & Diet Therapy	508	$ 4.00		**J. ART. COMPILATIONS** *(Cont'd.)*		
	Vol. 9 Community Health	509	4.00		Immunosuppressive Therapy Journal Art.	526	$20.00
	Vol.10 History & Law of Nursing	510	4.00		Institutional Laundry Journal Articles	789	8.00
	Vol.11 Fundamentals of Nursing	511	4.00		Lithium & Psychiatry Journal Articles	520	15.00
	Practical Nursing Examination Rev.- Vol.1	711	4.50		Outpatient Services Journal Articles	794	8.00
	MEDICAL OUTLINE SERIES				Psychosomatic Medicine Current J. Art.	788	12.00
	Cancer Chemotherapy	631	8.00		Selected Papers in Inhalation Therapy	523	10.00
	Otolaryngology	661	8.00		**TYPIST HANDBOOKS**		
	Psychiatry	621	8.00		Medical Typist's Guide for Hx & Phys.	976	4.50
	Urology	611	8.00		Radiology Typist Handbook	981	4.50
	CASE STUDY BOOKS				Surgical Typist Handbook	991	4.50
	Cutaneous Medicine Case Studies	014	7.00		**OTHER BOOKS**		
	ECG Case Studies	003	7.00		Acid Base Homeostasis	601	4.00
	Endocrinology Case Studies	008	10.00		Allergy Annual Review	325	12.00
	Gastroenterology Case Studies	004	10.00		Bailey & Love's Short Practice of Surgery	900	20.00
	Hematology Case Studies	020	10.00		Benign & Malignant Bladder Tumors	932	15.00
	Infectious Diseases Case Studies	011	7.00		Blood Groups	860	2.50
	Neurology Case Studies	006	10.00		Clinical Diagnostic Pearls	730	4.50
	Otolaryngology Case Studies	021	10.00		Concentrations of Solutions	602	3.00
	Pediatric Hematology Case Studies	018	10.00		Critical Care Manual	983	10.00
	Respiratory Care Case Studies	019	7.00		Cryogenics in Surgery	754	24.00
	Urology Case Studies	017	10.00		Diagnosis & Treatment of Breast Lesions	748	15.00
	SELF-ASSESSMENT BOOKS				English-Spanish Guide for Med. Personnel	721	2.50
	Self-Assess. Cur. Knldge - Nurse Anesthet.	715	7.00		Fundamental Orthopedics	603	4.50
	Self-Assess. Cur. Knldge - Infect. Diseases	263	10.00		Guide to Medical Reports	962	4.50
	Self-Assess. Cur. Knldge in Neurology	254	10.00		Handbook of Medical Emergencies	635	7.00
	Self-Assess. Cur. Knldge in Pathology	253	10.00		Human Anatomical Terminology	982	3.00
	Self-Assess. Cur. Knldge in Pediatrics	256	10.00		Illustrated Laboratory Techniques	919	10.00
	Self-Assess. Cur. Knldge in Psychiatry	252	10.00		Introduction to Blood Banking	975	8.00
	Self-Assess. Cur. Knldge in Rheumatology	258	10.00		Introduction to the Clinical History	729	3.00
	Self-Assess. Cur. Knldge in Surgery	250	10.00		Multilingual Guide for Medical Personnel	961	2.50
	S.A.C.K. Surgery for Family Physicians	259	10.00		Neoplasms of the Gastrointestinal Tract	736	20.00
	Self-Assess. Cur. Knldge in Urology	251	10.00		Neurology Handbook	604	8.00
	JOURNAL ARTICLE COMPILATIONS				Neurophysiology Study Guide	600	6.00
	Ambulance Service Journal Articles	517	10.00		Ophthalmology Rev. Essay Quest. & Ans.	347	10.00
	Blood Banking & Immunohemat. Jour. Art.	798	10.00		Outpatient Hemorrhoidectomy Lig. Tech.	752	12.50
	Emergency Room Journal Articles	795	8.00		Practical Points in Gastroenterology	733	7.00
	Hodgkin's Disease Journal Articles	515	12.00		Profiles in Surgery, Gynec. & Obstetrics	963	5.00
	Hosp. & Inst. Eng. & Maintenance J. Art.	793	8.00		Radiological Physics Exam. Review	486	10.00
	Hosp. Electronic Data Process. J. Art.	791	8.00		Skin, Heredity & Malignant Neoplasms	744	20.00
	Hosp. Housekeeping Journal Articles	790	8.00		Testicular Tumors	743	20.00
	Hosp. Pharmacy Journal Articles	799	10.00		Tissue Adhesives in Surgery	756	24.00
	Hosp. Security & Safety Journal Articles	796	8.00				
	Human Cytomegalovirus Journal Articles	522	15.00				

Prices subject to change